£15.54 AW
ATPEL

PAIN-FREE
ARTHRITIS

Web: ww
ter again

Also by Harris H. McIlwain, M.D.,
and Debra Fulghum Bruce, Ph.D.

Stop Osteoarthritis Now
Winning with Heart Attack
Winning with Back Pain
Winning with Chronic Pain
Winning with Osteoporosis
The 50+ Wellness Program
The Super Calcium Counter
The Unofficial Guide to Conquering Impotence
Bone Boosters
The Osteoporosis Cure
Super Aspirins
The Fibromyalgia Handbook

Also by Debra Fulgum Bruce, Ph.D.

The 24-Hour Turnaround
Miracle Touch
Overkill
The Sinus Cure
Making a Baby
Eat Right to Stay Young
The Snoring Cure
The Unofficial Guide to Impotence (Viagra)
The Unofficial Guide to Alternative Medicine
Breathe Right Now

PAIN-FREE ARTHRITIS

A 7-step program for feeling better again

Dr Harris H. McIlwain
and Debra Fulghum Bruce

PIATKUS

Copyright © 2003 by Dr Harris H. McIlwain and Debra Fulghum Bruce, Ph.D.

First published in the USA in 2003 by Henry Holt and Company LLC
115 West 18th St
New York, New York 10011

This edition first published in 2004 by Piatkus Books
Piatkus Books Ltd
5 Windmill Street, London W1T 2JA
email: info@piatkus.co.uk

The moral right of the author has been asserted

A catalogue record for this book is available from the British Library

ISBN 0 7499 2510 8

Text design by Victoria Hartman

This book has been printed on paper manufactured
with respect for the environment using wood from
managed sustainable resources

Data manipulation by Phoenix Photosetting, Chatham, Kent

Printed and bound in Great Britain by Antony Rowe Ltd, Chippenham, Wiltshire

Contents

Acknowledgments

We have received generous assistance, along with a wealth of reveal-ing testimony, from a select group of family, friends, and colleagues. We express our gratitude to the following: Robert G. Bruce, III; Michael Bockenek; Brittnye Bruce Bockenek, M.S.; Ashley Elizabeth Bruce; Claire Van Leuven Bruce, M.P.A.; Hugh H. Cruse, M.P.H, M.S./M.I.S.; Florence Leber; Laura E. McIlwain Cruse, M.D.; Kimberly McIlwain, M.D.; Michael McIlwain, D.M.D.; our medical illustrator, James Russell, M.S., for his excellent designs; Sunjay Daniel Trehan; and Christina Yarnoz.

Our agent, Denise Marcil, whose enthusiasm for this arthritis book boosted our motivation and creative prowess.

Our editor, Deborah Brody, for appreciation of an innovative holistic program for the treatment of arthritis and other pain-related problems.

Introduction

If you are among the 7 million people diagnosed with arthritis in the UK, and the tens of millions of sufferers around the world, you know the pain, stiffness, and outright misery it can cause. You can change that right now with this book!

Pain-Free Arthritis gives a proven 7-Step Program filled with workable solutions—natural and medical—that you can start immediately, as you finally get relief from debilitating and persistent pain caused by osteoarthritis, rheumatoid arthritis, fibromyalgia, carpal tunnel syndrome, and other pain-related problems. Unlike other books you may have read, *Pain-Free Arthritis* does not focus on one "cure" or remedy to end arthritis pain—there is no one cure that can do this. Rather, I give you a proven, tried-and-true holistic program that focuses on a wealth of alternative therapies, lifestyle changes, and medications to decrease pain and stiffness. This book was originally written for North American readers but the advice I give here applies to every arthritis sufferer, wherever they may live. UK information and statistics have been included where appropriate.

As a board-certified rheumatologist and geriatric medical specialist with Tampa Medical Group in Florida for the past twenty-five years, I've treated literally thousands of arthritis patients. Our group of rheumatologists has three pain clinics and an osteoporosis clinic that treat hundreds of patients each week. I'm also a certified medical director of long-term care facilities in Florida. Because I diagnose and treat pain-related diseases daily, I am passionate about finding ways to help my patients ease their symptoms.

While most patients rely on only medications to ease inflammation and pain, through years of research and professional experience I have discovered that there is much more to resolving arthritis pain than simply taking a drug. In *Pain-Free Arthritis*, you'll find a wealth of safe lifestyle substitutions, winning exercise and nutritional strategies, natural supplements and herbal therapies, mind/body and hands-on therapy tips, and fifty pain-free recipes. You'll also find information on the latest medications that have helped thousands of my patients resolve arthritis pain—*without* putting their active lives on hold.

The chances are that you are busy and want answers—*fast*—on how to reduce arthritis pain so you can continue being active and highly productive. Unlike other arthritis books, *Pain-Free Arthritis* places you at center stage by teaching you how a multifaceted program can help to resolve most types of arthritis pain. As you read through the steps in part I, and then on to the Recipes and Special Situations in parts II and III, you will see how the book gives you simple strategies to ease pain—with page after page of personalized self-help tips that you can use right now as you take control of your symptoms, stay healthy, and reduce your dependence on prescribed medications.

The Pain-Free Program is a medically proven lifestyle approach to permanently change the long-term prognosis of arthritis. It includes 7 basic steps that are scientifically substantiated, the result of my years of experience in helping thousands of patients to reclaim active lives in spite of arthritic conditions:

> Step 1: Start the Exercise Treatment
> Step 2: Follow the Pain-Free Nutritional Plan
> Step 3: Try Alternative Therapies
> Step 4: Make Key Lifestyle Changes
> Step 5: Consider Bodywork and Massage
> Step 6: Tap In to Pain-Free Mind Power
> Step 7: Choose the Latest Medical Treatments

The Pain-Free Program will guide you in setting exercise and diet goals, changing your lifestyle habits, monitoring your progress, and finding the right arthritis medication with the least side effects. This program guarantees to put you in control of your health—and arthritis—and covers a wide spectrum of strategies for the most common pain conditions.

Now that baby boomers are facing retirement years, pain treatment for arthritis is becoming even more important. In the United Kingdom, for example, the cost of drugs prescribed is about £341 million each year. More than half of all seniors suffer from pain; between 45 and 80 percent of long-term care facility residents are in pain. These statistics will only grow as we age and the number of arthritis cases increases because of our graying boomer population.

Pain is not healthy. You know how pain affects all aspects of life—your personality, concentration, productivity, sleep, relationships, eating habits, and overall health. New studies indicate pain may affect the immune system, so that cancer cells might speed up growth when there is pain in the body. Where does that leave the millions who have chronic arthritis pain every day? In this book, I'll show you how to wipe out pain and then manage the symptoms so arthritis does not rob your quality of life.

I know that your time is valuable. If you are like many of my patients, you're far too busy to sit down and read detailed medical information about arthritis. As one forty-six-year-old mother of three with osteoarthritis of the hands told me, "Dr. McIlwain, just tell me how to stop the pain. Life's too short for trial and error." The multitude of simple strategies in this program will do just that—show you how to stop pain and stop it quickly, so you can move on with your life.

Now, let's get started!

PART I

Pain-Free
Program

STEP 1

Start the Exercise Treatment

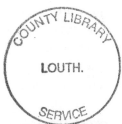

"Exercise? I can't even walk to the mailbox without pain." If you're like many of my patients, the thought of exercising is the furthest thing from your mind, especially if you have nursed chronic joint or muscle pain for months. Nevertheless, of all the treatment therapies for arthritis, exercise is the gold standard. Exercise gives the most guaranteed short- and long-term relief to end arthritis pain and stiffness. Not only does regular exercise boost all aspects of fitness, including strength, stamina, balance, posture, and overall coordination, it also increases circulation and keeps your bones and muscles strong and joints flexible.

Gather Your Pain-Free Tools

1. You'll need an inexpensive three-ringed notebook or your personal organiser to use as your Pain-Free Diary throughout the Pain-Free Program.
2. For Step 1, use the Pain-Free Diary to record your daily exercise regimen, including the time of exercise (morning or evening); type; duration; and how you felt before, during, and after exercise.
3. Write down how you feel after using moist heat applications twice each day. How does your pain feel after applications of ice packs? Refer to this as you decide on the best method for your pain.
4. Take the Pain-Free Diary to your next doctor's visit and discuss the feelings you have during and after exercise. Ask if medication changes might help you receive greater benefit from pain-free exercises that keep joints flexible and muscles strong.

Sam's Osteoarthritis of the Knee

Last year I consulted with Sam, a young attorney who could barely walk up the stairs because of chronic knee pain. A college athlete, Sam played minor league baseball for four years before attending law school. Now, at forty, Sam felt like a much older man. Because of injuries in early adulthood, his knees were stiff and achy. He had gained twenty pounds because he could no longer be active—and the added weight put more pressure on the already worn knee joint. After a physical examination and some tests, I told Sam of the diagnosis of osteoarthritis of the knee. I then explained that in osteoarthritis there is progressive loss of cartilage, the material that cushions the ends of bones, along with bony overgrowth. In addition, the tissue lining of the joint becomes inflamed, the ligaments get looser, and the muscles become weak—all resulting in pain when the joint is used.

Sam listened to all of this and then said, "Doctor, just tell me what I can do today to stop the pain, so I can enjoy my life again."

If only all my patients were like Sam, utterly willing to follow the pain-free suggestions I give to them! Because being active and exercise are important to me as an avid runner, I knew how important it was to Sam—and to other adults with arthritis—no matter what their age. I know what exercise can do to reduce stress, keep you well, help you maintain a normal weight—and reduce pain.

I discussed Step 1, "Start the Exercise Treatment," with Sam and promised that if he followed this step diligently, along with the six other pain-free steps, he'd see improvement within a few weeks and be able to play sports again. About three months later, I saw Sam and his young son at a professional hockey game. Sam sat near the top of the stadium, which meant he had walked many stairs with his injured, arthritic knee. He said that he follows the Pain-Free Program, and his knee pain had completely resolved. Sam had also lost about ten pounds, which has been shown to reduce pain in osteoarthritis, and was now riding bikes each evening with his son, working out at the gym during his lunch hour, and finally enjoying being an active young person again.

Sam's Exercise Treatment for Osteoarthritis

Before the Pain-Free Program

Exercise or Activity	Times per Week
1. Mowing the lawn	1
2. Swimming at the gym	2

After Beginning the Pain-Free Program

Exercise or Activity	Times per Week
1. Stationary bike	5
2. Biking with son	3
3. Swimming at the gym	3
4. Water aerobics class at the gym	4
5. Resistance exercise (strengthen knee muscles)	3
6. Stretches	7
7. Mowing lawn	1

Exercise: Your Arthritis Arsenal

Arthritis means inflammation in or around the joints that results in swelling, pain, and stiffness. It can generally be divided into two categories:

1. Osteoarthritis and other wear-and-tear types of arthritis
2. Inflammatory types of arthritis.

Most of the 100+ types of arthritis fall under each of these two categories. For instance, the most common types in the osteoarthritis group are the following:

- Osteoarthritis (OA)
- Fibromyalgia Syndrome (FMS)
- Bursitis/Tendonitis

While some types such as bursitis and tendonitis may not be thought of as arthritis per se, they mainly result from wear-and-tear changes. Likewise, in the inflammatory arthritis group, we have:

- Rheumatoid arthritis (RA)
- Arthritis with psoriasis (psoriatic arthritis)

- Ankylosing spondylitis
- Systemic lupus erythematosus (SLE or lupus)
- Gout (gouty arthritis)
- Pseudogout
- Polymyalgia Rheumatica (PMR)
- Infectious arthritis and Lyme disease

In all of these inflammatory types, the linings of the arthritic joints become inflamed, resulting in intense swelling, pain, and stiffness. (I've described the most common types of arthritis, including signs and symptoms, in appendix 2.)

No matter which type of arthritis, most people have pain, along with weakness in strength, flexibility, endurance, or exercise ability. In fact, for millions of people with arthritis, doing simple daily living tasks such as putting on clothes, tying shoelaces, combing hair, loading the dishwasher, or going out to get the mail can be painful.

Reduces Symptoms of Osteoarthritis

In our clinics, many patients tell how they simply avoid exercise altogether because of the anticipated added pain. However, a new study published in July 2002 in the journal *Arthritis and Rheumatism* confirms what I've been telling patients for two decades and what I'm telling you now: *If you don't move around and keep your muscles strong and joints flexible, your arthritis symptoms will worsen.* In this study, researchers evaluated 107 people with osteoarthritis of the knee and asked the participants to what degree they avoided activity during a painful arthritis flare. From the findings, researchers concluded that those people who avoided activity were more likely to be disabled than people who continued with undemanding activities or who took a break in between activities to make it through the day.

Reduces Symptoms of Inflammatory Arthritis

For those with inflammatory types of arthritis such as rheumatoid arthritis, exercise can give a tremendous benefit in easing pain, inflammation, and stiffness. In a revealing study published in the April 2002 issue of the *Annals of the Rheumatic Diseases*, researchers found that women with rheumatoid arthritis who had the thickest thigh muscles also had denser and stronger femurs (bone in the thigh). This finding supports the importance of exercise for women with rheumatoid arthritis in keeping muscles and bones strong and in preventing painful and debilitating fractures caused by osteoporosis, thinning of the bones. I might add that exercise is equally important for men, too, in staying strong and pain-free!

I diagnosed Pat with rheumatoid arthritis after she developed pain, stiffness, and swelling in her hands, wrists, knees, ankles, and feet. At first, this thirty-five-year-old computer technician thought the pain and other symptoms were from gardening, her weekend hobby. Yet, over a few months, Pat's symptoms didn't resolve, and she could no longer keep up with her workload because of the constant pain in her hands and wrists. Walking, standing, and even sitting at the computer work station became painful and limiting.

When I first saw Pat, she was considering reducing her hours at work or taking a medical leave because of the pain and fatigue. After examination and running some laboratory tests, I explained that she had rheumatoid arthritis, a common form of arthritis that causes inflammation in the lining (synovium) of the joints. With rheumatoid arthritis, the joint lining thickens, producing warmth, inflammation, and pain in the joint.

After prescribing medication, I immediately encouraged Pat to start the Exercise Treatment with twice-daily exercises, along with a whirlpool spa and warm showers for moist heat. Pat was determined not to let a chronic and painful illness rob her young life and started on the regular

Pat's Exercise Treatment for Rheumatoid Arthritis

Before the Pain-Free Program

Exercise or Activity	*Times per Week*
1. Walking (15 minutes)	3
2. Yard work	1

After Beginning the Pain-Free Program

Exercise or Activity	*Times per Week*
1. Range-of-motion exercises and stretching	6
2. Aquatics at the gym	3
3. Swimming in heated pool	3
4. Handheld weights	3
4. Gardening	2
5. Playing piano	7

use of moist heat and range-of-motion exercises, described below. After three weeks, Pat added 1-pound handheld weights and began working her muscles, using resistance. With medications and her exercise program, Pat noticed significant improvement in her pain and stiffness. After four months, she was almost back to her normal workload with little limitation by pain or stiffness.

Reduces Symptoms of Fibromyalgia

Exercise may also be the most effective treatment for those with fibromyalgia, as it helps to relieve deep muscle pain, chronic fatigue, and other exasperating symptoms. I've had fibromyalgia patients who were once unable to walk to their cars without excruciating muscle pain begin to enjoy pain-free walks around the neighborhood with friends after starting a regular exercise program. One patient, Janis, began teaching a low-impact water aerobics class at her fitness center only months after starting the Exercise Treatment. While many studies tout the benefits of exercise to those with arthritis, one study published in August 2001 in *Arthritis Care and Research* confirms that exercise is more effective than medication and alternative treatment at relieving pain and other symptoms of fibromyalgia. Another study published in the February 2002 issue of *Arthritis and Rheumatism* reiterated the same, as researchers found a regular program of resistance training and endurance exercise to be safe, well tolerated, and effective at improving muscle strength, cardiovascular endurance, and functional status in women with fibromyalgia yet without exacerbating symptoms.

Terri, age thirty-six, is an example of someone with fibromyalgia who reclaimed an active life after starting the Exercise Treatment. This young mother of twins had severe, limiting pain for three years, with all-over body pain, severe fatigue, and difficulty caring for her family. After her diagnosis of fibromyalgia, Terri began a program of twice-daily moist heat, using a shower or a heated pool, along with exercises, as outlined below. She also began walking on a treadmill for five minutes each day. Terri said she was embarrassed to tell anyone she could only walk for five minutes, especially when her friends all jogged for several miles each evening. I explained to Terri that she needed to do what was best for her body, and, with time, she would be walking longer distances. After a few weeks, Terri noticed increased flexibility and greater energy. She began to walk fifteen minutes daily and then joined an aquatics (water exercise) class at the gym.

Terri's Exercise Treatment for Fibromyalgia

Before the Pain-Free Program

Exercise or Activity	Times per Week
1. Daily housework	2
2. Watching twins play	7

After Beginning the Pain-Free Program

Exercise or Activity	Times per Week
1. Stretching exercises	7
2. Walking (20 minutes)	4
3. Swimming in heated pool	3
4. Aquatics at gym	3
5. Strength training	4
6. Playing with twins	7

Terri has continued to increase her exercises and has started weight training with supervision by the gym fitness trainer. I was especially pleased when Terri said that while she used to watch her twins play, she now actively plays with them. Because she is healthier and pain-free, her marriage is much stronger and her husband is grateful to have his "cheerful wife back." Terri is just one of many patients who has changed fibromyalgia from a severe, painful limitation to a manageable inconvenience.

Reduces Incidence of Disability

"If this works for my older sister and her hip pain, then these exercises may work for me." Sixty-eight-year-old Dolores and her seventy-four-year-old sister, Elaine, were both diagnosed with osteoarthritis of the hip. Elaine was diagnosed about a decade ago and was determined not to let arthritis ruin her retirement. As a retired schoolteacher, she did a lot of research on arthritis and immediately started a program of twice-daily moist heat, stretching and strengthening exercises, and medications to manage pain. Elaine claims that arthritis has not stopped her from being active, and she's able to do almost anything she wants—with no restrictions. While Dolores was recently diagnosed with osteoarthritis of the hip, she has seen the great success her older sister, Elaine, experienced with her pain-free exercise regimen and vows to follow the same.

Tim's Exercise Treatment for Rheumatoid Arthritis

Before the Pain-Free Program

Exercise or Activity	Times per Week
(Bedridden or housebound)	Full-time

After Beginning the Pain-Free Program

Exercise or Activity	Times per Week
1. Swimming	4
2. Water exercise	6
3. Stretches and range-of-motion exercise	6
4. Stationary bicycle	5
5. Walking at the mall	3
6. Yard work	3

I realize it's difficult to start exercising when you have joint or muscle pain, especially if you've lived a sedentary life for years. Nevertheless, a revealing study at Wake Forrest University School of Medicine found exercise to be a crucial factor in helping arthritis patients stay active each day. In this study published in October 2001 in the journal *Archives of Internal Medicine*, researchers confirmed that aerobic or resistance exercise appears to reduce the incidence of disability by about 50 percent in activities of daily living—meaning eating, dressing, using the toilet, or bathing. Although this study was performed on adults over age sixty, think of what these results mean to someone who is forty or fifty and just starting to notice the painful signs and symptoms of arthritis.

My patient Tim developed rheumatoid arthritis at age sixty-seven, only months after he retired as a successful real estate attorney. Unlike osteoarthritis, Tim's arthritis came on quickly with joint pain and stiffness upon awakening and rapid progression of pain and swelling in all of the joints of his arms and legs. For the first few weeks, he was severely limited to bed or a chair at home for any activity.

After the firm diagnosis of rheumatoid arthritis, Tim started a daily exercise program, along with medications and the twice-daily moist heat applications. At first, he was frustrated since the pain limited his exercise to just a few stretches in his swimming pool. However, Tim was determined to fight back. He continued the water exercise and after two weeks of daily stretches, he was able to swim two laps in the pool. In less than one month, Tim could swim twenty laps in the pool and ride a stationary bicycle for fifteen minutes during the evening news. His stiffness was greatly improved, and Tim started walking at the local mall with other friends. Within two months of starting his Exercise Treatment, Tim went on a planned weekend trip for a college reunion.

Strengthens Bones and Prevents Fractures

Exercise, particularly weight-bearing exercise, helps to keep bones strong and prevents osteoporosis. This is particularly important for women, as they begin to lose bone around age thirty-five, sometimes at a rate of 1 percent per year. During the immediate five- to ten-year period after menopause, which usually occurs around ages forty-five to fifty-five, this rate can increase to about 2 to 4 percent per year.

Walking, biking, dancing, aerobics, and other weight-bearing exercises stimulate the cells that make new bone. By increasing weight-bearing exercises, we encourage our bodies to form more bone and can delay or actually reverse the destructive process of osteoporosis that results in painful or debilitating fractures. By adding strength training, you improve your muscle strength and flexibility, and reduce the likelihood of falling as you get older.

Beth's exercise program actually helped her to return to work. This sixty-one-year-old grandmother and bookkeeper was bothered for years by chronic pain in her lower back from osteoarthritis, but she continued to work long hours to help support her grandson, who lived with her. When I first saw Beth, she had severe pain in her middle and lower back and had stopped work because the pain prevented sitting and standing for more than a few minutes at a time. X rays showed that in addition to her osteoarthritis, Beth had osteoporosis and several fractures in the vertebrae of the spine. In osteoporosis, the bones become thinner than normal and break more easily.

Immediately, Beth started medications to increase bone density and prevent future fractures. She also started twice-daily warm showers to ease her back pain and stiffness, along with stretching, range-of-motion exercises, and strengthening exercises. She slowly increased the exercises as her pain subsided, and within a few weeks, Beth was walking on her treadmill in the morning and riding bikes in the evenings with her teenage grandson. Just eight weeks after beginning the Pain-Free Program, Beth returned to work and was able to work a full day.

Beth's back exercise program achieves two goals:

1. It strengthens the back muscles to give more support to the spine and nearby soft tissues, resulting in much less pain.
2. It helps to increase the bone density in the spine, helping to prevent future painful fractures.

Beth's Exercise Treatment for Osteoporosis

Before the Pain-Free Program

Exercise or Activity	Times per Week
1. Housework	2
2. Sitting at desk at work	5

After Beginning the Pain-Free Program

Exercise or Activity	Times per Week
1. Range-of-motion and stretching exercise	5
2. Strengthening exercise with weights	5
3. Walking on treadmill	4
4. Swimming at the gym	2
5. Housework	3
6. Working full-time	5
7. Riding bike with her grandson	7

Boosts Endorphins and Mood

There are still more benefits of exercise for those with arthritis. Regular exercise produces alpha waves in the brain that are tied to feelings of serenity and are prominent during relaxation. Exercise reduces anxiety and stress and might improve mood in those with depression. Exercise also releases endorphins, which are brain chemicals that are natural mood elevators. Almost all of my patients who exercise regularly experience improved sleep. Healing sleep is vital for those with chronic illnesses, as medications often interfere with deep sleep, leaving you feeling lethargic, fatigued, and even depressed. In fact, there are studies discussed in the chapter on Step 4 that link sleep loss with a decrease in the body's pain threshold, causing arthritis symptoms to flare. You can gain control of these symptoms by following the 7-Step Program, beginning with your Exercise Treatment.

10 Exercise Benefits

1. Keeps muscles strong and joints limber.
2. Builds endurance and strengthens the cardiovascular system.
3. Boosts bone density to prevent fractures.
4. Sharpens reaction time and helps decrease risk of falls. Exercise boosts oxygen to the brain, which is then sent to your muscles.
5. Lowers blood pressure and heart rate.
6. Improves mood and helps sleep.
7. Burns fat and helps to maintain a normal weight.
8. Helps reduce the risk of diabetes mellitus.
9. Relieves tension and helps keep you alert.
10. Increases self-image.

Increases Physical Activity and Life Span

If you think exercise is for the young, think again. My patient Betty, age ninety, is enjoying her life more than many people half her age. Betty has osteoarthritis and osteoporosis in the spine, which can be extremely painful and makes it difficult to be active. But Betty has found that the more active she is, including exercise, the less pain she feels, and the less medication she needs.

Betty uses her exercise bike daily for twenty minutes and does strengthening exercises with hand weights—sometimes combining the two exercises to get a full body workout. When arthritis patients tell me, "I'm too old to exercise," I always tell them about Betty and remind them that age may be, in part, in their minds.

Recent findings in the May issue of the *Journal of the American Medical Association* (*JAMA*) discussed a landmark study in which researchers interviewed and followed more than 15,000 people from 1977 through 1994. In this experiment, researchers found that leisure-time physical activity is associated with reduced death even after genetic and other family-related factors are taken into account. No matter what your age, if you start Step 1, the Exercise Treatment, now, you will feel relief of nagging pain and be on the road to preserving your ability to be active for years to come.

Three Rules for Pain-free Living

Before you start any exercise program, always check with your doctor to make sure you can gradually begin a program. Ask if there are any restrictions on exercise or activity, and see which type of exercise will give your arthritis the greatest benefits. Also, if you are taking medications, discuss these with your physician before starting your Exercise Treatment. Some medications interfere with heart rate and blood pressure and may affect the way you feel during exercise. Also, be sure to follow these three rules as you begin your program:

Rule 1: Use Moist Heat or Ice Applications

Use warm, moist compresses on the arthritic joint or painful muscle for fifteen minutes before exercise. Moist heat dilates blood vessels and increases the flow of blood, oxygen, and nutrients to the painful site. You may use a moist heating pad or a warm, damp towel. You can also stand or sit on a stool in the shower and let warm water hit the painful area on your body. It may help your stiffness to use the moist heat for a few minutes after exercising.

Some patients prefer ice packs, which reduce swelling and pain by constricting blood vessels. You might try a bag of frozen vegetables or ice wrapped in a clean towel. Apply this to the painful joint or muscle for 10 to 15 minutes at a time. There is some new research published in the March 2002 issue of the *Journal of Rheumatology* indicating that ice packs may help with some forms of arthritis, such as gout. In the study, researchers gave both groups of participants prednisone and colchicine, common treatments for acute gout attacks. One group also received ice-pack therapy while the other group did not. Researchers found that patients who received ice packs had significant reduction in pain compared with the patients who did not have this therapy. While medications are necessary to treat gout, more studies will help to confirm these results. This study does show how natural therapies may be helpful in some conditions to lessen symptoms and perhaps allow you to take fewer medications.

Alternating moist heat applications with ice packs may bring optimal relief. The most important thing is to find the pain-relieving therapy that works best for you, and make this your daily ritual before and after exercise.

Rule 2: Balance Exercise with Rest Periods
After working out, most people with arthritis have some discomfort. Usually these symptoms will improve after applications of moist heat, a warm bath, or an ice pack and rest. If your pain takes longer than normal to improve, give yourself an added rest period, perhaps an extra 24 hours, to increase healing. Then begin exercise again after using moist heat, but start with fewer repetitions this time and follow up with moist heat immediately. Avoid resting for longer than 24 hours since it can cause more stiffness in the joint and add to muscle weakness.

Rule 3: Stop if Your Pain Worsens
If your pain becomes severe during exercise, stop until you check with your doctor or physical therapist. If you feel only slight discomfort, but you can continue exercise, try a few repetitions and gradually build as you can. If you have pain for more than 20 minutes after exercising, you probably did too much. It would be wise to start with fewer repetitions next time and then slowly increase, as long as your pain is not increasing. For example, decrease to 2 or 3 repetitions, and when you can do these comfortably, increase to 4 repetitions. Add another repetition when you can master one level without pain, and then increase accordingly.

At times when your joints are swollen and inflamed some types of exercises may not be helpful. So, talk to your doctor before you start any exercise program to make sure it will benefit your type of arthritis. Always balance exercise with rest during flare-ups.

Your Arthritis Arsenal

To receive immediate benefits from your Pain-Free Program, in the Exercise Treatment incorporate a variety of daily exercises, including the following:

- Stretching at least 10 minutes daily, including the specific range-of-motion exercises beginning on page 266.
- Biking, swimming, walking, or other aerobic exercise, starting with as little as 1 minute or less daily and gradually working up to your goal of 30 minutes, five times a week.
- Strengthening exercise, weight lifting, or resistance machines (if approved by your doctor), including the isometric exercises on page

267. Start with 1 minute and gradually work up to 10 to 15 minutes, three times a week.
- Gardening, housecleaning, or other similar activities daily.

Stretches

Stretches are range-of-motion exercises that reduce stiffness and help keep your joints flexible, which can make daily activities easier. Simply put, your "range of motion" is the amount your joints can move in each direction. If you don't regularly flex your muscles and move your joints through their full range of motion, your muscles will become shorter and tight. The good news is that most middle-aged and older adults can become just as flexible as young adults, if they stretch regularly.

Benefits: Slow, gentle stretches gradually expand your range of motion, giving you greater flexibility, less arthritis pain, and improvement in overall function, which helps to reduce the chance for falls and injuries. Although there is some debate in the medical community about the need to stretch before exercise, some new findings reinforce the belief that pre-workout stretching can help to prevent injury. In a study presented at the Experimental Biology 2002 Conference, investigators reported that injury-preventing immune system inflammatory cells called neutrophils were seen in large numbers among the passive-stretching muscle fibers. It is thought that these neutrophils have a protective effect on the muscle, helping to block injury during exercise. Researchers confirmed that passive stretching before exercise protects the muscle from injury.

Risks: Make sure you've warmed up by walking around for a few minutes before stretching to keep your tendons flexible and increase blood flow to the muscles.

Bottom line: Stretching and range-of-motion exercises help to relieve stiffness and keep joints flexible.

Exercise Treatment: Your stretching routine should be specific and include all the major muscle groups, including the shoulders, hips, pelvis, buttocks, thighs, and calves. Carefully move to the maximum range of motion of the joint that you are able to do easily, without pain or unusual discomfort. Then slightly increase the motion until you feel resistance or discomfort. Do this only once. When you can do this range of motion with no pain or discomfort, try it twice. As you gradually increase (with no pain or discomfort), you may find that flexibility increases.

- For stretches: Start with the basic stretches on page 263, 2 or 3 minutes daily. Work up to 10 minutes each day for maximum pain relief. Make sure your muscles are warm (after exercise or physical activity) before you begin your stretches.
- For range-of-motion exercises: Start with the range-of-motion exercises on page 266. Go slowly with 1 or 2 repetitions, and increase to 15 to 20 repetitions of each exercise, twice daily.

GOOD CHOICES FOR ARTHRITIS
Stretching
Range-of-motion exercises

Strengthening or Resistance Exercise

Strengthening or resistance exercise is anaerobic, meaning without oxygen, and forces the body to work its muscles against an object of resistance. By using free weights, machines, or even your body's weight as resistance, you can strengthen the muscles and bone, decrease body fat, and improve your endurance and ability to perform daily tasks with less threat of injury or falls. Just as aerobic or conditioning exercise strengthens the heart by challenging it to adapt to the stress of exercise, weight training challenges muscles and bones to adapt to the stress of resistance and forces them to become stronger.

Resistance exercise helps to keep muscles strong so they can bear the stress on your joints. When you avoid exercise, the muscles become weak and cannot support the body's weight. This results in increased pressure on joints, as well as added pain and stiffness. Resistance exercise strengthens muscles, helping to keep bones strong, which prevents bone loss, osteoporosis, and fractures.

Benefits: A study conducted at Tufts University found that people with rheumatoid arthritis could safely increase their strength by up to 60 percent with a modest training program. Another study, published in the *Journal of the American Medical Association,* also found improvements in osteoarthritis when patients combined weight training with aerobic exercise. To gain the strengthening benefit without irritating the joints, proper technique is important so as not to cause further injury.

Risks: Strength training may not be right for your type of arthritis, so talk to your doctor or rheumatologist before you start. If you do try a strengthening exercise and your muscles begin to hurt, wait several days for your pain to resolve before doing it again. If you have arthritis in the hands, shoulders, or neck, avoid working with free weights since this may put added pressure on your joints. Also, avoid holding your breath while lifting weights since it can cause a great increase in blood pressure. (Exhaling during the lift and breathing easy during the exercise can prevent this.)

Bottom line: Be sure to check with your physician, and then it would be helpful to talk with a physical therapist so that you have a program planned with your special needs in mind. In addition, age is *no* factor with weight training; the muscles of older people can remain almost as responsive as the muscles of younger people. While some older adults may not be concerned with building muscle, strength training is an excellent way to help prevent falls—stronger muscles keep your body balanced and flexible.

Exercise Treatment: Start with a weight you can easily lift ten times with the last two repetitions being increasingly difficult. A weight that becomes difficult at eight repetitions has been shown in studies to be an effective stimulus for strengthening and toning muscles. For some people the weights are only 1 to 2 pounds; others can start at 15 to 20 pounds, depending on their muscle strength and arthritic condition. As your muscles gain strength and if there is no additional pain, increase the weights in 1- to 2-pound increments.

With your strengthening workout, you should work your arms and shoulders, abdomen, chest, back, and legs. Do each lift slowly to get maximum benefit, and aim for 10 to 15 minutes, three times a week. Studies show that you only need to do one set of the exercise to derive benefit. Doing more sets may fatigue the muscle and may even defeat your purpose.

GOOD CHOICES FOR ARTHRITIS
Isometric rope
Elastic bands
Swim gloves and kickboard, using the water as resistance
Hand iron gloves*
Free weights
Resistance machines

---

*Hand iron gloves are weight gloves (1 to 3 pounds for each hand) that are safer for the wrists than holding dumbbells or handheld free weights.

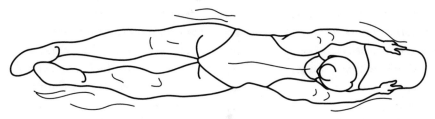

Figure 1.2.

Kickboarding.

Weight Training Helps to Burn Fat

Muscle mass is metabolically active tissue and burns calories. The more muscle mass your body has, the more calories you burn all day. Fat burns 2 to 3 calories per pound while muscle burns 50 calories per pound.

Endurance or Aerobic Exercise

Aerobic exercise means "with oxygen" and includes activities that use the large muscles of the body in repetitive or rhythmic motions. Aerobic exercise improves the cardiovascular system and overall health, and benefits weight control, mood, and general health. Examples of aerobic exercise are walking, swimming, dance, aquatics, bicycling, or exercising on treadmills or rowing machines. Daily activities such as mowing the lawn, raking leaves, sweeping the driveway, playing golf, or walking the dog are also aerobic exercise.

Benefits: Aerobic exercise is a great benefit for weight control—an important risk factor for some types of arthritis. Did you know that if you lost just ten pounds, you might reduce the pain of osteoarthritis of the knee by up to 90 percent? Exercise is the best way to drop those ten pounds and prevent many types of arthritis as you keep your joints moving in their range of motion.

Risks: If you overexercise, your joints may become inflamed and stiff. If your exercise causes pain that lasts for more than 20 to 30 minutes or leaves you feeling unusually fatigued, cut back on your exercise regimen. Start again at a lower level, and gradually increase.

Bottom line: According to the American College of Rheumatology, 20- to 30-minute exercise routines can be performed in increments of 10 minutes over the course of a day. Use moderate exertion with your aerobic or conditioning exercise. This means that during exercise you can speak normally and are not out of breath. If you become overheated or have difficulty speaking, slow down until your body feels comfortable again. If you have severe or unusual pain, stop until you can consult your doctor.

Exercise Treatment: Do moderate-intensity aerobic exercises for a few minutes and gradually increase to 20 to 30 minutes at least three days a week. Or, do mini-workouts—short, 10-minute periods of aerobic activity that you do throughout the day. These include a 10-minute walk on the treadmill or around the block, a 10-minute burst on your stationary bike, or even vacuuming, washing windows, or parking your car at the end of the lot and walking to your destination, if you do so actively. Mini-workouts may be far more effective for those with arthritis, as they are conveniently implemented in your daily routine and help to keep joints limber and muscles strong.

GOOD CHOICES FOR ARTHRITIS

Aquatics*	Stair machine
Biking	Stationary bike
Dancing	Swimming
Gazelle Freestyle Glider (see box)	Tai chi
Low-impact aerobics	Treadmill
Mini-workouts	Walking
Rowing machine	

Try a Heated Pool for Ease in Movement

If you have trouble starting exercises because of pain, exercise in a whirlpool, warm bath, heated pool, or warm shower. The moist heat will make it easier to move the joints with much less pain and stiffness.

---

*Aquatics consist of exercises done in a warm-water pool. In water, you are buoyant and are relieved of about 80 to 90 percent of your body weight, allowing you to move around but without stress on your joints. Water provides 12 to 14 percent more resistance than air, making aquatics an excellent resistance workout, too.

The Gazelle Freestyle Glider

I discovered the Gazelle Freestyle Glider cross-training workout machine after several patients brought me literature and asked my opinion. After doing some research and then purchasing one for my home fitness room, I realized that the freestyle range-of-motion design helps you to receive a cardiovascular, resistance, and stretching workout—all at one time. What makes this piece of equipment beneficial for those with arthritis is there is no added pressure on the ankles, feet, knees, or hips as with pounding on pavement during walking. The Gazelle Freestyle Glider or similar equipment is available at most sporting goods stores, department stores, and online distributors. It is a machine that you can use in the privacy of your home for an "all in one" low-impact aerobic, stretching, and resistance workout. In a standing position, you place your feet in the respective gliders and then carefully hold on to the handlebars. Then, starting slowly with a "push and pull" arm movement, you stretch your arms and legs and move them back and forth, as if you were cross-country skiing, yet you fully control the aerobic pace and effort.

Five Pain-Free Workouts to Do Anytime

1. *Internet Isometrics.* Place a small tennis ball under your foot while sitting at the computer. Roll your foot over the ball, using the muscles in the foot and ankle. Doing this regularly can help to strengthen the ankle and decrease pain and stiffness.
2. *TV Aerobics.* Keep the remote control on top of the TV, so you have to get up to change channels manually when watching favorite shows. If you are a habitual channel surfer, this mini-workout will be even more effective for you!
3. *Back Strengthener.* Push your chair away from your computer terminal or desk. Reaching your hands in front of you, lock your fingers with your palms turned outward. Keeping your back straight and posture upright, extend your hands as far from your body as possible. Now gently turn your shoulders to the right, continuing to keep your arms out in front, and then return to the original position. Gently turn your shoulders to the left, and return to the original position. Repeat this stretch five times to each side, and try to do it periodically throughout your day.

4. *Traffic Strengtheners.* Keep a foam exercise ball in your car, and use this to keep hands and wrists nimble while waiting in lines of rush-hour traffic. Squeeze with opposite hands to loosen finger joints and relax wrist muscles.

5. *Desk Stretches.* At work or in a long meeting, practice the rules of good posture. Practice holding your stomach muscles in while pulling your shoulders back to align your posture. Relax your shoulders, and let your head roll forward with your chin to your chest. Gently rotate your head in a circle. Repeat five times. Rotate your head in the opposite direction, and repeat five times. Be careful not to strain your neck.

Pain-Free Strategies

Pain-Free Strategy #1: Count during exercise. Counting, either to yourself or aloud, during exercise may help you reach your goal without getting bored. A good rule of thumb is that walking 2,000 steps equals one mile; 1,000 steps equals a half-mile. Counting also distracts you so you do not mentally focus on pain you may feel. Distraction is an excellent mind-body therapy that helps diminish the pain you feel while you wait for the arthritis medication to kick in.

Pain-Free Strategy #2: Start a combination exercise program. Combining the three types of exercise in your pain-free regimen will give you the most benefit. A good example of this benefit is discussed in the February 2002 issue of the journal *Arthritis Care and Research*. In the study, researchers show how a combination program of strength training and walking (aerobic exercise) reduces fibromyalgia symptoms in just weeks.

Pain-Free Strategy #3: Consider purchasing a whirlpool spa to ease pain before and after exercise. Heat is a vasodilator that increases blood flow and helps to decrease inflammation and pain; moist heat, such as from a Jacuzzi or other whirlpool, is the most effective way to apply this natural pain relief—and it easily fits into your active lifestyle. It may even be tax deductible if you doctor writes a prescription for it. A whirlpool attachment for your bathtub is also available. Ask your doctor—and your CPA—to make sure.

Daily Living Activities Count as Exercise

Not only does exercise include biking or stretching, but there are a host of daily activities that count as exercise, such as raking leaves, working in your garden, sewing or knitting, or playing the piano, if you have arthritis of the hands. All of these activities help to keep your muscles strong and joints working in their full range of motion.

Examples of Moderate Amounts of Daily Activity

- Dancing
- Gardening
- Mowing the lawn
- Playing actively with children or grandchildren
- Pushing a stroller
- Raking leaves
- Running
- Stair walking
- Walking the dog
- Washing and waxing a car
- Washing windows or floors
- Wheeling self in wheelchair

For Women Only

If you're a middle-aged woman, you may notice more aches and pains than before. According to the federally funded *Women Across America* study, middle-aged women often have significant difficulty climbing a flight of stairs, carrying groceries, or even walking around the block because of a decrease in muscle and increase in body fat. This loss in muscle mass is known as *sarcopenia,* and it is a factor in the occurrence of frailty and likelihood of falls as we age. When you combine muscle loss with arthritis, which usually happens around the same time, you are at increased risk of injuries—if you don't get in control with your Exercise Treatment.

Start Your Exercise Treatment

Using the information in this chapter, you can begin to develop a personalized physical activity and exercise program that can help you to feel relief from unending arthritis pain. However, no matter what your initial commitment, *consistency* is the key to feeling optimal relief with your Exercise Treatment. This means you must stick with your program on good and bad days—even on days when you don't "feel" like exercising. The more the exercise and physical activities become a part of your daily life, the sooner you will achieve pain-free living.

Treatment 1: Set Pain-Free Goals. You cannot control the fact that you have arthritis. Nevertheless, you *can* control how you manage the pain and stiffness. Make sure that the exercise goals you set are specific so you can measure your progress. Also, make sure that the goals are realistic as you attempt a program you can actually achieve. For instance, if you start your Exercise Treatment by riding a stationary bike, set a goal of 2 to 5 minutes daily for the first week. Once you do this successfully, as you can, add another 1 to 2 minutes to your daily regimen until you reach the level you wish to achieve. Avoid setting your goals too high at first, as you might stop your program altogether. If you have more pain for 20 to 30 minutes after you exercise, reduce the length of the next workout.

Some suggested goals include the following:

- I'll talk to my doctor before starting the Exercise Treatment.
- I'll take my prescribed medication daily.
- I'll start with the stretching exercises and use moist heat applications before and after stretches.
- I'll walk (or bike) for 5 minutes each morning.
- I'll add more exercises as I feel stronger.
- I'll cut back when I feel increased pain or fatigue.
- I'll stick with the Exercise Treatment, even when I don't feel motivated.

Treatment 2: Find Exercises and Physical Activities You Enjoy. To stay consistent with your Exercise Treatment, you have to find exercises and physical activities that you enjoy. Review the range-of-motion and isometric exercises starting on page 266, along with the lists of exercises in this step. Record those that appeal to you in each category. Be sure to read the Doctor's Treatment at the end of this step to make sure the exercises you choose are helpful for your type of arthritis. If in doubt, check with your doctor or a physical therapist.

Treatment 3: Schedule a Daily Exercise Time. Whether you choose to walk, bike, or swim, it's important that you choose some type of physical activity daily to keep your muscles strong and joints flexible. Doing the

My Exercise and Activity List

Stretches	Strengthening Exercises	Aerobic Exercise	Daily Physical Activities

suggested range-of-motion and isometric exercises during or immediately after your morning shower or warm bath may help you to feel less pain and be more flexible and active throughout the day. Once you establish a certain exercise time, stick with it. Schedule this time in your daily calendar, and don't let anything—or anyone—divert your attention. Remind family members that exercise will help you to feel better, so you can gain their support. During inclement weather, make sure you have a backup plan for indoor exercise such as a stretching video, riding a stationary bicycle, or walking on a treadmill or at a nearby mall.

Fill in the following Exercise Treatment:

My Exercise Treatment

Before the Pain-Free Program

Exercise or Activity   *Times per Week*

1.
2.
3.

After the Pain-Free Program

Exercise or Activity   *Times per Week*

1.
2.
3.
4.

Treatment 4: Keep an Exercise Log. Many patients find it helpful to keep an exercise log, in which they record specific goals and chart daily progress. You can use the Pain-Free Diary (see page 3) or a large calendar.

Sample Weekly Exercise Log

Day of Week	Type of Exercise	Time of Day	Duration	Feelings During	Feelings After	Medication
Monday	Stretching	7 A.M.	10 minutes	Stiff	Sore	NSAIDs*
	Stretching	7 P.M.	10 minutes	Sore	Sore	
Tuesday	Aquatics	9 A.M.	20 minutes	No pain	Achy	NSAIDs
	Stretching	7 P.M.	10 minutes	Stiff	Sore	
Wednesday	Stretching	7 A.M.	10 minutes	No pain	No pain	NSAIDs
	Stationary bike	6 P.M.	10 minutes	Stiff	Achy	
Thursday	Stretching class	9 A.M.	20 minutes	Stiff	No pain	NSAIDs
Friday	Stretching	7 A.M.	10 minutes	No pain	No pain	NSAIDs
	Swimming at gym	5 P.M.	20 minutes	No pain	No pain	
Saturday	Stretching	7 A.M.	10 minutes	No pain	No pain	NSAIDs
	Gardening	9 A.M.	30 minutes	No pain	Stiff, achy	
Sunday	Stretching	7 A.M.	10 minutes	Stiff	No pain	NSAIDs
	Walking	3 P.M.	20 minutes	No pain	No pain	

*NSAIDs are nonsteroid anti-inflammatory drugs.

Be sure you write down the type of exercise, the time of day, the duration, and how you felt during and after exercise. Record any medications you are taking, too. If you have any new pain, write this down so you can share with your doctor.

Treatment 5: Exercise with a Group. If your exercise compliance is low, you might consider exercising with a group. Check with your local gym or contact your local support group for classes in your area. Some patients walk after work with friends in their neighborhoods. Others enjoy walking at the mall with local support groups.

Doctor's Exercise Treatment

Osteoarthritis (OA)
OA of the Knee
- Start with bike-riding outdoors or use an indoor stationary bike to strengthen the muscles of the thighs (the quadriceps in front; the hamstring muscles behind). Strengthening these muscles will give support for the knees and help to reduce pain. Use low resistance when you first start biking, making sure it's easy to pedal without too much pain. Start with a few minutes each day and gradually

---

Let's Review: 8 Steps
to Getting Started with the Exercise Treatment

1. Talk to your doctor for approval to start regular exercise. Stay on your prescribed medications.
2. Use a warm shower or other moist heat applications to loosen stiff joints or sore muscles before exercise.
3. Warm up by walking or jogging in place, moving your limbs at the same time. Gradually increase the warm-up until your heart rate and body temperature are elevated.
4. If you are new to exercise or haven't worked out in a while, start with the slow, gentle stretches and range-of-motion exercises on page 263. Go easy at first with just a few repetitions, and build as you gain strength.
5. Add an aerobic exercise, listed on page 20, as you progress. You may do the aerobic exercise for 3 to 5 minutes at first. Do what feels comfortable to you, and stop if you feel tired or experience more pain.
6. Once you can comfortably do the stretching and aerobic exercises, start the strengthening exercise, using light weights (1–2 pounds) at first. Increase the weight as you are able. Again, even a few minutes of resistance exercise will help you build muscle strength. Increase this time, as you get stronger.
7. Have a cool-down period after the exercise period, using slow, gentle stretches.
8. Use moist heat or cold packs on sore muscles and stiff joints immediately following exercise. Continue the Exercise Treatment and increase your daily activities as you become stronger and pain-free.

---

increase your time, as you feel stronger. If you have pain after biking, reduce the length of time for your next session or stop altogether.

- If biking is too painful, do the knee exercises starting on page 275. Then add strengthening exercises by using a few pounds of weights (or resistance) to the knee exercises.
- Check out an exercise program for arthritis at your local gym. A local support group may be able to guide you.

OA of the Hip
- Start with the range-of-motion exercises on page 266.
- Start riding an exercise bike. Go slowly with low resistance and gradually increase, as long as there is no pain.

- Focus on the back and knee exercises, pages 270 and 275, as stronger back muscles will help strengthen and support the hips.
- Check with your local gym for aquatic exercise programs. Your local support group can also suggest programs near you.

OA of the Hands

- Start with exercises on page 277, which help build flexibility and strength. Use a soft foam ball (not a hard tennis ball) to exercise your handgrip and to increase dexterity. Use activities such as knitting or playing the piano to keep your fingers nimble and reduce pain.

OA of the Shoulder

- Do the shoulder exercises on page 268 while taking a warm shower. The moist heat will allow you greater movement and less pain. Also, check out aquatics classes at your local gym. Swim laps in a heated pool, starting slowly as you work to build strength in the shoulder muscles and increase flexibility in the joint.

OA of the Spine

- For the back and neck, start with the exercises on page 266. Gradually increase to 20 repetitions, and then add resistance or light weights with the guidance of a fitness trainer or physical therapist.
- Try swimming for a few minutes a day, gradually increasing your swim to about 30 minutes several times each week.

OA of the Ankles/Feet

- Start with the exercises on page 275 to strengthen the muscles of the legs for ankle and foot support. Talk to a fitness instructor at the gym. There are specific resistance machines that can greatly strengthen the legs and ankles, but use these only with the help of a trainer.

Fibromyalgia (FMS)

- Start with stretches, page 263, and do these every morning after a warm shower or bath.
- Follow with the range-of-motion exercises on page 266, and work up to 20 repetitions of each exercise. It may take weeks or even a few months to see real benefit. Once you are stronger and have

reduced pain, increase your exercise program. The more exercises you do, the better you will feel.

- After you can do 20 repetitions of the range-of-motion exercises, start resistance exercises, explained on page 17. Most FMS patients find that working with a personal trainer or physical therapist helps to reduce the chance of injury.
- Increase exercise, as you are able, adding walking, swimming, or an exercise bicycle. Water exercise or aquatics at your local gym in a heated pool may be helpful since these activities eliminate weight on painful muscles. Try to do water exercise in the late afternoon to help induce restful sleep at night.

Carpal Tunnel Syndrome

- Avoid repetitive use of the wrist, such as constant typing on a computer keyboard. A wrist splint can help prevent too much activity, which can greatly aggravate your symptoms.
- Once your carpal tunnel symptoms are controlled, take time throughout your day to stretch the arms, wrist, and fingers to protect them from injury.

Bursitis and Tendonitis

- Follow the specific exercises on page 266 for the site involved, using moist heat before and after exercise. If you still have no relief, ask your doctor about medication or a local injection.
- Rest the elbow or other site involved until pain becomes controlled. Follow the specific exercises for tennis elbow, page 274, or other sites involved to prevent future attacks.
- Talk to your doctor about medication or a local injection, which may help if you don't have rapid improvement.

Rheumatoid Arthritis (and Other Inflammatory Arthritis)

- Stretching and range-of-motion exercises (see page 266) should be used for all arthritic joints. Start with 1 or 2 repetitions of each range-of-motion exercise and gradually increase until you can do 20 repetitions. Be sure to use moist heat baths or applications before and after exercise to reduce pain and stiffness. When you can do 20 repetitions, add strengthening exercises, including the isometric exercises on page 267.

- Consider swimming, which is a great way to work all the joints, as well as the back. Start with 1 to 2 minutes in a heated pool, and slowly build to a goal of about 30 minutes a day, which can be divided into 10-minute segments. Even if you can do only a few exercises or a few minutes using a kickboard, start somewhere. Increase the exercise or laps each exercise period until you work up to your goal time. You can always supplement swimming with other exercises, such as bike riding or strengthening exercises. Don't let the fact that you have arthritis stop you from exercising the way you wish. However, you may benefit from a trainer or therapist who can personalize your exercise program and help you to avoid injury.

Gout

- Avoid exercise during a gout attack. Instead, rest the painful joint. (The pain can be so severe that nothing else is possible!) Talk to your doctor about medications that can shorten the attack. Apply ice packs to the painful joint for added relief (see page 14).

Follow the Pain-Free Nutritional Plan

What if you could turn *off* your arthritis pain and stiffness simply by eating a certain food? With all the new nutritional research, this idea is not far-fetched, and someday food may be the medicine of choice for those with arthritis and related diseases.

In Step 1 you identified specific exercises that will help you decrease pain and increase mobility and learned that moist heat treatments before and after exercise can give you optimal relief. The next step of your Pain-Free Program will help you to evaluate your current diet and eliminate those foods that might trigger arthritis symptoms; increase healing foods to reduce inflammation and pain; and lose weight. In fact, your body weight is an accurate predictor of how much pain you might feel. It's my clinical experience that people who are 20 percent or more over their normal body weight have greater problems with their arthritis than those who are at a normal weight.

Set Your Pain-Free Weight Goal

Oftentimes in our clinics, patients ask if there is some food they can eat to cure their arthritis. They bring in newspaper or magazine clippings with the latest food cures designed to help reduce arthritis pain and stiffness. One young mother with rheumatoid arthritis said her aunt recommended that she drink apple cider vinegar before each meal and gargle with it at bedtime to keep her joints well lubricated. I wish it were that simple!

Living a pain-free life with arthritis takes time and energy. In addition, there is no strong scientific data that one food can cure this painful

---

Gather Your Pain-Free Tools

1. Use your Pain-Free Diary (see page 3) to record your daily food intake.
2. If you start the weight-loss plan, you'll need a measuring tape to record your measurements before and during the diet. Measure your chest, waist, hips, and thighs, and record these measurements in your Pain-Free Diary every two weeks.
3. You need access to accurate scales to measure your weight before and during the weight-loss plan. Weigh before starting the Pain-Free Diet and record this. Then weigh every two weeks at the same time of day, and record this in your diary.
4. You need an inexpensive calorie-counting guide or access to the United States Department of Agriculture website for nutritional information (http://www.nal.usda.gov/fnic/foodcomp/Data/). At this site, you can download the nutritional content of most common foods or search the database online.

---

disease. However, one of the most important actions you can take right now is to maintain a normal weight. For some patients, maintaining an ideal weight gives the most improvement in pain, stiffness, and mobility. In our clinics, I've seen men and women lose ten to thirty pounds and suddenly regain their ability to exercise and live very active lives.

"What's the best weight for me, Doctor?" Almost every patient asks that question when I mention that shedding a few pounds could very well alleviate arthritis pain and allow them to cut back on medications. You don't have to lose a lot of weight to experience tremendous relief from pain and gain increased mobility. In fact, because of body mechanics, dropping only ten pounds will take a thirty-pound load off your hips and knees and could decrease your risk of knee osteoarthritis by almost 50 percent.

While height-weight charts used to give an accurate range, newer studies show that your body mass index (BMI) seems to give a more accurate picture of health. BMI is defined as body weight (in kilograms) divided by your height (in meters) squared. New studies show that as defined by body mass index, one of every two British adults is overweight or obese.

The BMI number, or value, correlates to your risk of adverse effects on health, with higher numbers showing an increased risk. According to the American Dietetic Association, people with a higher percentage of body fat tend to have a higher BMI than those who have a greater percentage of muscle. It is this extra body fat, not muscle, which puts you at greater risk for health problems.

Here's how to figure out your BMI:

1. Write down your weight in pounds _____.
2. Multiply that number by 703 (____ × 703) = _____.
3. Multiply your height in inches by itself (___ × ___) = _____.
4. Divide the figure in number 2 by the figure in number 3 to get your BMI _____.

Comprehensive research reveals that maintaining a normal body weight is important for staying well and avoiding chronic illness such as diabetes or heart disease.

Staying at a normal weight may also play a role in the pain you feel. In a study published in the March 2002 issue of the *Scandinavian Journal of Rheumatology*, investigators concluded that weight loss might improve physical functioning in those with fibromyalgia. In the study, researchers compared FMS symptoms at different levels of BMI and found that the higher the BMI, the greater the symptoms of fatigue and painful trigger points.

BMI Categories

BMI	*Category*
19 or less	Underweight
20–25	Acceptable weight
26–30	Overweight
31 or more	Obese

Arthritis 101

Did you know that weighing just ten to fifteen extra pounds puts you at high risk of osteoarthritis of the knees, hip, and spine? OA strikes the weight-bearing joints, so the higher the weight, the more wear and tear on your joints. Experts estimate that each extra pound you gain is equal to two to three additional pounds of stress on your knees. Want to avoid this chronic pain? Follow the weight-loss instructions in this key step of the Pain-Free Program.

Lose Weight to Reduce Pain

Caroline, a fifty-two-year-old bank executive, couldn't believe that losing just ten pounds would give her dramatic relief from osteoarthritis knee pain. "I've avoided exercise for two years because I was so afraid of having more pain. I'd take the elevator instead of the stairs and even used the valet service at the bank to avoid walking across the parking lot.

"But after losing ten pounds, I cut back my medications to just one nonsteroidal anti-inflammatory drug daily. I now walk stairs, ride my bicycle, and even play tennis with my husband. The weight loss made all the difference in letting me be active again."

Even if you are five or ten pounds over your normal weight, dropping these extra pounds is important for your joints and overall health. Excess pounds put extra strain on knees, hips, and other weight-bearing joints, not to mention your heart! Being overweight or obese actually worsens the joints—making them stiffer and more painful, and can exacerbate arthritis flares.

Calories In + Calories Out = Weight Loss

No matter what the fad-diet gurus claim, losing weight is a simple mathematical equation; that is, to lose weight you must burn more calories (energy) than you ingest. I realize this is often a catch-22 for those with arthritis, as it's hard to lose weight if you can't move around because of severe joint or muscle pain and stiffness. Many sedentary patients claim to stay on a low-calorie diet without weight-loss success simply because they are unable to be active. I hope after reading Step 1, you will reconsider your current lifestyle and, along with the Pain-Free Nutrition Plan, start the Exercise Treatment—to lose weight, decrease pain, and increase mobility.

You need at least 1,200 calories daily to have adequate energy for the body while still losing weight. Many case studies demonstrate that severely restricting calories (less than 1,200) diminishes metabolism and keeps you from maintaining the weight loss. When your diet is too low in calories, your body's metabolism slows down to conserve body fuel and needs fewer calories. This can result in no weight loss at all—even though you are eating very little food.

The American Dietetic Association recommends a calorie level of *no less than ten times your desired weight*, with women getting at least 1,200 calories and men getting at least 1,400 calories per day. This daily calorie allowance will not allow a quick reduction of weight, but studies show that it is better to make lifestyle changes and lose weight slowly to make the adjustment less stressful. Gradual behavior modification is more likely to be successful, especially in terms of keeping your weight under control. To estimate how many calories you need daily to lose weight, use the following formula:

Multiply your ideal weight in pounds by 10
10×140 (ideal weight) = 1,400 calories
10×170 (ideal weight) = 1,700 calories

For example, a woman who wants to weigh 140 pounds needs 1,400 calories daily; a man who wants to reach 170 pounds needs 1,700 calories daily. Of course, if you are extremely active, you may eat more calories than this and still experience weight loss. If you are extremely sedentary talk to your doctor or a registered dietitian about your caloric intake needed for weight loss.

Assess Your Energy Outflow
Once you've calculated the necessary daily calories to lose weight, realistically look at your energy expenditure, in exercise and daily activity. The amount of calories (or energy) you burn during exercise depends on your weight, the activity, and the intensity level at which you're performing the exercise. If you are a sedentary person, then make plans to incorporate more activities in your daily routine. You can maximize your weight loss and receive a pain-free benefit for joints and muscles by being more active. Use the following list as a guide:

Activity	*Calories burned per hour per pound body weight*
Bicycling, 10 mph	2.6
Dancing, modern	2.6
Golf, walking	2.3
Hiking	3.6
Rowing machine	3.1
Skiing, downhill	2.6
Swimming, slow crawl	3.5
Walking, 3.5 mph	2.4
Weight training	1.9

Keep a Daily Diet Log

Use the Pain-Free Diary to keep track of your progress. Write down your current weight, clothes size, and waist measurement, along with the goals you hope to accomplish. Every two weeks, record this information again. If you are not experiencing a decrease in weight, clothes size, or body measurements, then reevaluate your diet and exercise plan to see if you need to make some changes.

Keep a record of food intake. Log everything in the diary, including meals, desserts, sweets, chewing gum, and those small "tastes" during food preparation (you'll be surprised at how this adds up!). All calories are equal when it comes to losing weight, and staying within your daily calorie allotment is important in reaching your goal.

Review your daily diet log each evening. Look for destructive patterns. For instance, if you find yourself eating more at a certain time of day, plan ways to overcome this habit, such as avoiding the kitchen or food preparation at those times or eating in another room and using a smaller plate. If you overeat while watching television, fix a small bowl of plain popcorn or plate of chopped celery and carrots to quench your need to munch. Or if you find that you sample everyone's food as you clean the dinner plates, chew sugar-free flavored gum, which will help cut the urge to eat prepared foods. (One of the nurses at our clinic swears by sugar-free grape bubblegum to keep her from snacking.)

Karen, a fibromyalgia patient who lost almost eighty pounds over a period of eighteen months, said she brushed her teeth frequently throughout the day to avoid eating snacks. "It was hard to think of eating snacks when my mouth had a strong wintergreen flavor from my toothpaste. If I found myself losing control and eating more, I simply brushed my teeth and then used handheld mouthwash sprays, which I kept in my kitchen, desk and purse."

Whatever it takes to revamp your eating habits, do it. Find simple solutions that help you to avoid snacking and overeating at mealtimes and you will gain confidence in meeting your weight-loss goals—as well as reap the ultimate reward of less pain and increased ability to exercise and be active.

Select Foods Low on the Glycemic Index

If you've failed to lose weight following the standard low-fat, high-carbohydrate diet that has been touted as healthy, there may be good reason. Some intriguing studies on the glycemic index (GI), a rating system that ranks foods on how they affect our blood sugar levels, confirm that foods high on the GI (mostly carbohydrates such as potatoes, rice, pasta, and breads) increase blood sugar and insulin levels. Then, after a few hours, these chemicals fall rapidly and trigger symptoms of hunger and weakness. Yet, foods low on the GI (vegetables, certain fruits, and lentils) keep blood sugar and insulin levels even, helping to increase fullness for longer periods.

The glycemic index was originally intended for diabetics. Now, some researchers believe that the popular low-fat, high-carbohydrate diet may be counterproductive to weight control because it markedly produces a high glycemic response, promoting body-fat gain. In contrast, diets based on low-fat foods that produce a low glycemic response (low-GI foods) may enhance weight control because they promote satiety, minimize insulin secretion, and maintain insulin sensitivity. Thus, this diabetic diet may help healthy adults to lose weight when low-fat, high-carb diets have failed.

Using the chart below, select foods for your meals that are at the low end of the glycemic index, such as yogurt, soy, fruit, vegetables, and lentils. Be selective when eating foods higher on the GI such as white bread, potatoes, pasta, and desserts. Always stay within your estimated calorie range for weight loss when choosing any food.

A low GI lunch:	Salad with cheese, chicken, and ham; sliced apple
A medium GI lunch:	Whole-wheat spaghetti and meat sauce with coleslaw
A high GI lunch:	Bagel with cream cheese, banana, and butter cookies

The Glycemic Index

Food	Glycemic Index
Baked potato	135 (High end)
Cornflakes	119
White bread	100
Wholemeal bread	99
Brown rice	96
Raisins	93
White rice	83

Banana (raw)	79
All-Bran	73
Sweet potato	70
Spaghetti (white)	66
Spaghetti (wholemeal)	61
Baked beans	60
Ice cream, yogurt, whole milk, apple	49–53
Red lentils	43
Soy beans	20 (Low end)

Use Portion Control

No matter what eating plan you choose, portion sizes can make or break a weight reduction program. You can be on target with the right foods for weight reduction, but if you eat too many of these foods, you have sabotaged your goal of losing weight. An understanding of portion size is crucial to see a significant reduction in your weight. Check out the following to estimate a serving size. Another tip is to keep servings about the size of the palm of your hand.

Measure Servings

Bread, Cereal, Rice, and Pasta

1 slice of bread (wholegrain and pumpernickel are better choices)
½ hamburger bun (1 bun = 2 portions)
½ bagel (1 whole bagel = 2 portions)
½ English muffin
½ large pita or flat bread
¾ ounce or 20g of pretzels
½ cup or 100g cooked cereal, pasta, or rice
¾ cup or 100g of unsweetened dry cereal

Fruit

1 medium-size piece of fruit
¾ cup or 100g berries
1 cup or 170g melon chunks
½ cup or 50g grapes
½ cup or 90g chopped, cooked, or canned fruit
½ cup or 120ml fruit juice
¼ cup or 60ml nectar

Vegetables
½ cup or 90g cooked greens
1 cup or 30g raw greens (spinach, cos lettuce, and more)
1 cup raw or 120g cut-up vegetables (broccoli, cauliflower, and more)
½ cup or 80g cooked cut-up vegetables (broccoli, cauliflower, and more)
1 carrot
2 stalks celery

Milk
1 cup or 240ml skim milk
1 cup or 240ml fat-free, sugar-free yogurt
1 ounce or 30g cheese
¼ cup or 4 tablespoons fat-free or reduced-fat cottage cheese
1 cup or 240ml reduced-fat soymilk

Meat and Meat Substitutes
1 ounce or 30g cooked low-fat beef, pork, poultry, or fish
½ chicken breast
2 slices of roast beef (3 × 3 × ¼-inch thick)
½ to 1 cup or 80–170g cooked beans
¾ cup or 150g flaked fish
2 eggs
½ cup or 120ml low-cholesterol egg alternative

Legumes and Soy Products
½ cup or 60g soy nuts
½ cup or 80g cooked beans or lentils (black beans, kidney beans, and more)
3 ounces or 80g tofu
3 ounces or 80g tempeh

Fats
1 teaspoon vegetable oil or margarine
1 tablespoon salad dressing
3 teaspoons seeds or nuts
⅛ medium avocado
10 small or 5 large olives

Eat Frequently
It's interesting that when most people decide to lose weight, they immediately start dieting and stop eating. Dietitians say the best way to

lose pounds and maintain a normal weight is to stop dieting and eat more frequently with smaller meals. Dieting can often be hazardous to your health, since it restricts calories and nutritious foods, causing feelings of deprivation and often resulting in rebound binging or overeating. I believe life gives us enough obstacles—such as arthritis joint or muscle pain—than to create one more by withholding food.

When I tell patients to eat more frequently to lose weight, they sometimes misunderstand. For instance, one patient took me literally and ate every few hours—but she ate a liberal four-course meal each time. Imagine how upset she was when she had gained eight pounds by her next office visit! I now fully explain the reasoning and studies behind this theory, that researchers have found that people who eat two meals or less during the day have a slower metabolic rate (the speed at which your body burns calories, and the rate that we all want to go faster) versus those who eat three or more times a day. Eating frequently will also keep your blood glucose constant so you won't feel irritable or overly hungry.

An easy way to adjust to mini-meals is to break your daily food intake into five or six small meals. Space these meals every three to four hours throughout the day. Each mini-meal will have about 200 to 300 calories, depending on your total caloric goal. Your daily menu may look similar to this:

Sample Daily Diet of Mini-Meals

Mini-Meal	Food Choices	Calories
1. Breakfast	1 slice whole grain bread, omelet with egg substitute, 1 cup or 240ml skim or soy milk, coffee	300
2. Snack	1 cup or 240ml lite or soy yogurt, ½ cup or 60g berries	150
3. Lunch	3 ounces or 80g water-packed tuna (drained), 1 tablespoon low-fat mayo, lettuce, tomato, 2 slices whole grain bread, 1 apple, water with lemon	400
4. Snack	2 cream crackers, 1 tablespoon peanut butter, ½ cup or 120ml skim or soy milk	200
5. Dinner	3 ounces baked skinless chicken breast, 1 cup steamed broccoli, ½ cup cooked carrots, 2 cups field greens salad with flavored vinaigrette, mineral water	300
6. Snack	3 cups air-popped popcorn, ½ cup red grapes	150
Total Calories		1,500

Boost Healing Nutrients in Your Diet

There are some new studies on nutrients that may be important for boosting wellness, particularly for those who must take powerful arthritis medications. For instance, a study published in July 2001 in the journal *Arthritis and Rheumatism* confirmed that taking folic acid or folate supplements along with methotrexate, a commonly prescribed medication for rheumatoid arthritis, can help to decrease drug-related liver damage. This key nutrient may allow rheumatoid arthritis patients to stay on the medication longer and benefit from relief of pain and inflammation without the medication's deleterious side effects. Dietary folate gives the same benefit, and later on in this step I will explain which foods are high in this nutrient.

Choose Whole Foods

Food is the most important source of natural vitamins, minerals, antioxidants, phytonutrients, and fiber. While vitamin manufacturers would like you to think that the natural dietary supplement gives you the same benefit as eating the real thing, that's not totally true. Food has nutrients that we have not yet identified that are important in bolstering optimal health. That's why I encourage patients to first eat a healthy, well-balanced diet to meet their dietary requirements and to focus on whole foods instead of those that are prepackaged or processed. However, if you can't eat a balanced diet or if you are taking medications, then be sure to take a good multivitamin/mineral supplement.

Supplement or Not?

The recommended daily allowances (RDAs) are established by the National Academy of Sciences and National Research Council as the amount necessary to prevent gross deficiency syndromes. It has become apparent to many experts that these levels are not adequate for all people, especially for older adults or those with chronic diseases. Many times a chronic illness can put you at higher risk for nutrient deficiencies as you ingest lower levels of vitamins and minerals, and medications often wreak havoc with the body. For example, some of my rheumatoid patients often show deficiencies in vitamin C, D, E, calcium, and folic acid. Likewise, those patients with osteoporosis are sometimes deficient in vitamin D and calcium. Arthritis patients who take corticosteroids to reduce arthritis inflammation should consider calcium supplements to make sure they will not suffer bone loss—a side effect of long-term steroid treatment.

Different Types of Supplements

- *Time-released* supplements dissolve slowly in the intestine over a six-
  to twelve-hour period, thus increasing the absorption of a vitamin or
  mineral.
- *Chelated* minerals are designed to increase absorption in the body.
- *Superpotency* or *therapeutic* supplements contain at least one
  ingredient in a dose ten times or more greater than the RDA
  (Recommended Daily Allowance).

If you need supplementation in your diet, follow these safe suggestions:

1. Start with a multiple vitamin that has the Recommended Daily
   Allowance as suggested by the American Dietetics Association.
2. Consult a State Registered Dietitian (S.R.D.) about your specific
   vitamin and mineral needs. Take into consideration your age,
   current health status, type of arthritis, and medications.
3. Ask your doctor to recommend a safe vitamin/mineral supplement. But keep in mind that a vitamin/mineral supplement is just
   that—a supplement to your regular, healthy diet. I recommend
   checking out the "Silver" and "Over 50" formulas because the
   mineral levels are usually appropriate for most people.

Include Healing Foods

A host of studies reveal the benefits of certain foods and nutrients in
reducing symptoms of arthritis and related diseases. Use the following
information to assess your daily diet and include these nutrient-dense
foods in your meal plan, as you continue your pain-free goals:

Vitamin C May Prevent the Progression of Osteoarthritis
Scientists have long noted that vitamin C (otherwise known as ascorbic
acid) plays a key role in building and protecting collagen, an important
part of the cartilage, which cushions the joints as they move. In
osteoarthritis, the cartilage wears away and becomes less efficient in its
job of cushioning the joint.

As an antioxidant, vitamin C protects DNA from free radical damage,
helps to control inflammation, and plays a part in rebuilding and
regenerating damaged joint tissue. Some new findings suggest that

vitamin C may also help prevent the progression of osteoarthritis. In the Framingham Osteoarthritis Cohort Study, part of the fifty-year Framingham Heart Study on residents in Framingham, Massachusetts, participants with osteoarthritis of the knee who had a higher intake of vitamin C also had a reduced risk of cartilage loss and disease progression. In this study, fifty-nine arthritis patients took ascorbic acid (300–1,000 milligrams per day). Researchers found that abnormal capillary fragility improved, as well as improvement of pain and other symptoms. While more studies will confirm if vitamin C can halt or slow the progression of osteoarthritis, this study gives some promise of a nutritional connection.

Vitamin C also helps to boost levels of the energizing brain chemical norepinephrine, which produces a feeling of alertness and increases concentration. This is especially important for those with fibromyalgia who experience periods of inattentiveness or "fibro fog."

Pain-Free Treatment: 500 to 1,000 milligrams (mg). You can get 90 milligrams of vitamin C by eating five servings of fresh fruits and vegetables daily. Eat plenty of broccoli, cauliflower, peppers, kale, Brussels sprouts, cabbage, citrus fruit, melons, berries, fruit juices, asparagus, avocado, tomato, and watercress.

Vitamin B$_3$ May Improve Joint Flexibility

When it comes to improving joint flexibility, vitamin B$_3$—also called niacin or nicotinic acid and niacinamide or nicotinamide—may bring some relief. New National Institutes of Health research has linked vitamin B$_3$ with improved joint range of motion and reduced pain and swelling. The report, published in the July 1996 issue of *Inflammatory Research*, concluded that niacinamide improved joint flexibility, reduced inflammation, and allowed for reduction in standard anti-inflammatory medications when compared to placebo. In another similar study published in October 1999 in *Medical Hypothesis*, researchers concluded the same: nontoxic nutritional therapies, such as niacinamide, may prove beneficial in preventing and halting osteoarthritis with enhancing glucocorticoid secretion.

Most people get ample vitamin B$_3$ in their diets from foods such as yeast, peanut butter, potatoes, and rice. Niacinamide, the form of vitamin B$_3$ used in the study, is usually safe to take, although rare liver problems have occurred at doses in excess of 1,000 milligrams per day.

Pain-Free Treatment: 15 to 20 milligrams. Eat plenty of Brewer's yeast, wheat germ, enriched breads, mushrooms, green vegetables, peanut butter, potatoes, and rice. Talk with a registered nutritionist if supplementation is needed.

Vitamin B_6 May Ease Carpal Tunnel Pain

It's hard to get through daily activities when you have carpal tunnel syndrome. Many of my patients who worked with computers considered changing careers because the chronic pain and numbness interfered with their work. However, some new findings give hope, suggesting that vitamin B_6 deficiency may cause an increased susceptibility to carpal tunnel pain and numbness. Vitamin B_6, a water-soluble vitamin, is important for the synthesis of serotonin and dopamine, neurotransmitters that are necessary for healthy nerve cell communication.

Pain-Free Treatment: 50 milligrams. In order to avoid vitamin B_6 deficiency, make sure to eat foods that contain this important nutrient on a daily basis. If you do supplement, the Institute of Medicine of the National Academies of Science recently established 100 milligrams of vitamin B_6 as the upper limit. Vitamin B_6 is one of the few water-soluble vitamins that may be toxic if taken in large doses. Taking too much may cause nerve damage to the arms and legs.

Eat plenty of chicken, fish, liver, kidney, pork, bananas, spinach, sweet potatoes, potatoes, chickpeas, walnuts, brown rice, soybeans, sunflower seeds, avocado, oats, peanuts, lima beans, peanut butter, prunes, and whole-wheat products.

Folic Acid Counteracts Drug-Related Liver Disease

New research continues to give us a better understanding of the link between food and arthritis. In a study published in the July 2001 issue of *Arthritis and Rheumatism*, researchers show that folic acid may help to counteract drug-related liver damage in those with rheumatoid arthritis, an autoimmune disease that often strikes people in their thirties and forties. The illness causes the immune system to attack tissues that line the joints, which can cause pain, inflammation, and joint destruction. In the study, researchers confirmed that taking folic acid or folate supplements along with methotrexate, a commonly prescribed medication for rheumatoid arthritis, could help to decrease drug-related liver damage. This allows patients to stay on the medication longer and see greater relief of pain and inflammation. Dietary folate may give the same benefit.

Another reason to get ample folate, through food or supplementation, is to improve your mood. Research shows a high incidence of folate deficiency in depression, and clinical studies indicate that some depressed patients who are folate deficient respond to folate administration.

Pain-Free Treatment: 400 micrograms (mcg) or 0.4 milligrams. If you need to supplement, the risk of toxicity is low. Eat plenty of fortified breakfast cereals, wheat germ, spinach, oranges, broccoli, asparagus, beetroot, spinach, cabbage, egg yolks, turkey, chickpeas, lentils, black beans, kidney beans, and soybeans. (The doses most commonly used as a supplement in rheumatoid arthritis are 1 milligram daily in the USA, and 5milligrams daily in the UK.)

Pantothenic Acid May Ease Arthritis Symptoms

You probably know people who take Brewer's yeast and claim that it helps them to feel energetic. Nevertheless, could this supplement high in B vitamins work to ease pain for those with arthritis? Some new evidence says yes. Research suggests that people with rheumatoid arthritis (RA) may be partially deficient in pantothenic acid (vitamin B_5). In one placebo-controlled trial, those with RA had less morning stiffness, disability, and pain when they took 2,000 milligrams of pantothenic acid per day.

Pain-Free Treatment: 500 milligrams. Although many doctors suggest therapeutic doses of pantothenic acid (sometimes as high as 2,000 milligrams for those with rheumatoid arthritis), the studies are not conclusive. Stick with your daily vitamin and mineral tablet to ensure getting adequate amounts of pantothenic acid, along with other necessary nutrients.

Eat plenty of Brewer's yeast, whole grain breads and cereals, dried beans, avocados, fish, chicken, liver, nuts (pecans, hazelnuts), peanuts, cauliflower, mushrooms, potatoes, oranges, bananas, milk, cheese, and eggs.

Vitamin D Keeps Bones Strong

To build bone and keep bones strong through the years, calcium must have special "boosters" to help it absorb efficiently in the body. Vitamin D, a fat-soluble vitamin also known as calciferol, is one such booster. Although this vitamin is found in some foods, such as vitamin D-fortified milk, most of the vitamin D used for strong bones comes from sunshine.

While calcium metabolism in the body is dependent on vitamin D, this vitamin also plays a role in the normal turnover of articular cartilage. In a prospective study of 556 participants in the Framingham Heart Study, low dietary intake of vitamin D and low serum levels of the vitamin were each associated with increased progression of osteoarthritis of the knee. In the study, those who ate a diet high in vitamin D or who took vitamin D supplements had a 75 percent reduction in the risk of their arthritis progressing. This study suggests adequate intake of vitamin D may slow the progression and possibly help prevent the development of osteoarthritis.

Taking a 15 to 20-minute walk outside several times a week should keep your body well supplied with enough vitamin D to keep bones healthy. Some studies show that because vitamin D is fat soluble, it can store in the body. This means that casual exposure to sunlight in the summer months may allow your body to have ample amounts of this vitamin in the winter. However, for those who work in offices year-round, exposure to sunlight through windowpane glass may result in vitamin D deficiency.

Vitamin D has similar actions to a hormone in the body since it helps activate calcium and phosphorus into the bloodstream. Not only are these two minerals necessary for strong bones, they are also important in keeping muscles and nerves healthy. When the body has an insufficient supply of vitamin D, the blood levels of calcium and phosphorus drop as well. Where does the body turn to get more of these much-needed minerals? You guessed it—your bones. Loss of the minerals calcium and phosphorus is directly related to osteoporosis and a host of other bone-weakening problems.

Pain-Free Treatment: 400 International Units (IU). If you are over fifty, talk with your doctor about the need for vitamin D supplements. Along with sunlight, you can also obtain this vitamin from food sources, such as halibut-liver oil, herring, cod-liver oil, mackerel, salmon, tuna, fortified margarines, and fortified cereals. There are 400 IUs of vitamin D in most multivitamin supplements.

Vitamin E May Fight Arthritis Damage
Vitamin E may be key to fighting arthritis-like damage. In a comprehensive study published in March 2002 in the journal *Arthritis and Rheumatism*, French scientists reported that vitamin E reduces joint destruction in mice with a rheumatoid-like arthritis. In humans, experts believe the rheumatoid arthritis patients have low blood levels of antioxidants, such as vitamin E and C, which are necessary to fight the destructive effects of free radicals, potentially damaging by-products of the body's metabolism. The French investigators found that after six

weeks of vitamin E treatment, the arthritic mice had less severe bone and cartilage destruction than that in animals that did not receive vitamin E. Whether this remains to be true in humans is still under investigation. However, I believe studies like this show the tremendous value of a healthy diet in keeping us disease- and pain-free.

Pain-Free Treatment: 400 to 800 International Units (IUs). Eat plenty of cold-pressed seed and nut oils, wheat germ, nuts, mango, pumpkin, and green leafy vegetables like broccoli, spinach, and spring greens. You can also find vitamin E in meat, fish, poultry, clams, mackerel, lobster, salmon, and prawns. The health risk of too much vitamin E supplementation is low, although there are a few studies on long-term supplementation. The Institute of Medicine has set the upper tolerable limit for vitamin E supplementation at 1,500 IUs (1,000 mg) as bleeding may occur at higher levels.

Vitamin K
Vitamin K is an essential nutrient in bone mineralization. Low levels of vitamin K have been found in people with osteoporosis-related fractures. In addition, studies indicate that low levels of circulating vitamin K are associated with low bone density.

Pain-Free Treatment: 65 to 85 micrograms (mcg). Eat plenty of broccoli and other cruciferous vegetables, rapeseed oil, soybean oil, bran, beef liver, and olive oil.

Boron May Help Ease Osteoarthritis
Boron has only recently been recognized as an essential trace element for plants, but has only recently been considered possibly essential for humans. In Australia, where much of the food is grown on soil deficient in this mineral, it's reported that boron supplements were popular as a treatment for osteoarthritis. These supplements started to sell at a rate of 10,000 bottles per month before the Australian government took the boron products off the market. An interesting study on boron comes from Austria where twenty people were randomly assigned to receive boron (6 milligrams per day) or a placebo for eight weeks. Fifty percent of those patients who took boron experienced improvement compared with only 10 percent of those taking a placebo. There were no reported side effects, and researchers concluded that boron supplementation may be helpful for individuals with osteoarthritis whose diets are low in this mineral.

Most people get adequate amounts of boron in their daily food intake. If your diet is limited, make sure your daily multiple vitamin and mineral supplement contains boron.

Pain-Free Treatment: There is no established recommendation for boron intake. Eat plenty of iron-enriched cereals and breads, fruits, vegetables, legumes (dried beans and peas), dried fruits, leafy greens, nuts, and seeds.

Calcium Keeps Bones Strong

Calcium is a mineral that helps build strong bones and teeth. During childhood and young adult years, calcium helps to build strong bones. Later in life, calcium helps to keep bones strong and prevent osteoporosis. About 91 percent of the body's calcium stores are in the bones and teeth; 1 percent is in the soft tissue and blood. If you do not ingest calcium, the body will take the calcium it needs from the body's stores. After a period of time, you will get osteoporosis because the chronic lack of calcium causes the bones to become weak and less dense. There are many foods high in calcium, including fortified soy products, which are also low in fat.

For those who do not get ample calcium through food, calcium supplements are effective in boosting the body's source of this mineral. In many studies, calcium citrate is found to dissolve more easily than carbonate or phosphate, and it is bioavailable, meaning your body can use more of what you ingest. If you take calcium supplements, be sure to follow these rules:

- Avoid taking more than 500 milligrams of calcium at once.
- Take supplements with food for best absorption.
- Do not take supplements with high-fat or high-fiber foods, as these foods interfere with the absorption of calcium.
- Do not take calcium supplements with foods high in iron.

Pain-Free Treatment: Eat plenty of broccoli, bok choy, salmon, sardines with bones, kale, beans (dried), dairy products, fortified soy products, and calcium-fortified foods. (See chart: "Recommended Calcium Intakes.")

Magnesium Eases Fibromyalgia Symptoms

In those with fibromyalgia, magnesium appears to inhibit nerve receptors linked to the trigger point pain and regulate the release of neurohormones. In a new study published in the March 2002 issue of *Alternative*

Recommended Calcium Intakes*

Ages	Amount Mg/Day
Birth–6 months	210
6 months–1 year	270
1–3	500
4–8	800
9–13	1,300
14–18	1,300
19–30	1,000
31–50	1,000*
51–70	1,200*
70 or older	1,200*
Pregnant; lactating	1,000
14–18	1,300
19–50	1,000

Source: National Academy of Sciences (NAS)
*I recommend that postmenopausal women take in a total of 1,500 mg calcium each day between diet and supplements.

Bone-Building Greens (per Half-Cup Serving)

Vegetable	Calcium Content
Spinach	122 mg
Endive	90 mg
Kale	46 mg
Broccoli	31 mg
Watercress	20 mg
Rocket	16 mg

Medicine Alert, researchers found that an oral dose of 500 milligrams a day of magnesium significantly increases muscle magnesium level and influences fibromyalgia symptoms. (Side effects of magnesium supplements may include gastrointestinal symptoms and diarrhea.)

Magnesium therapy should be administered with a doctor's supervision. Talk to your doctor and see if this supplement can be combined with your medical treatment to help lessen muscle pain.

Pain-Free Treatment: 500 to 750 milligrams. Dietary magnesium does not present a health risk, but there are risks with taking too much of magnesium supplements. Eat plenty of cereal, nuts, sunflower seeds, tofu, diary products, bananas, pineapples, plantains, raisins, artichokes, avocados, lima beans, spinach, okra, beet greens, hummus, oysters, halibut, mackerel, grouper, cod, and sole. You can get magnesium in your daily diet by using various herbs, including coriander, dill, celery seed, sage, dried mustard, basil, cumin, tarragon, marjoram, and poppy seed.

Phosphorus Helps to Form Bone

Phosphorus and calcium work hand in hand in forming new bone. Because of the interaction between the two elements, in individuals with diets low in phosphorus, calcium supplementation alone is inadequate and, in fact, can aggravate an existing phosphorus deficiency. As a result, a calcium phosphate product may be preferable in women undergoing bone-building therapy, according to a new study presented at the recent National Osteoporosis Foundation Symposium in Honolulu.

Pain-Free Treatment: 1,200 milligrams. Eat plenty of lean meat, fish, nuts, beans, dairy products, breads, cereals, and other grain products.

Selenium Keeps Immune System Functioning

Selenium is a trace mineral that may hold the key to staying disease-free because it helps to keep the immune system working optimally and is important for a healthy thyroid gland. Selenium is an important part of the antioxidant enzyme because it helps to fight free radicals that cause damage to healthy tissue.

There are some studies on rheumatoid arthritis patients indicating that they have reduced selenium levels in their blood. This may be because these people have a low intake of selenium through foods (see "Food Sources of Pain-Free Minerals" below). Current findings are preliminary and no recommendations for selenium supplements are available.

Pain-Free Treatment: 200 micrograms daily. Eat plenty of Brazil nuts, beef, tuna, turkey, chicken, walnuts, cheese, eggs, cottage cheese, and enriched grain products. A 3½-ounce or 100g serving of tuna gives you a full day's requirement of selenium.

Zinc Is Necessary for Bone Health

Zinc is an essential mineral for good health, keeping your immune system actively fighting viruses and bacteria and helping to support healthy growth and development. For osteoporosis prevention, zinc is also crucial since it enhances mineral absorption and is essential for bone health.

Pain-Free Treatment: 15 to 50 milligrams daily. Eat plenty of meat, pork, poultry, seafood, wheat products, nuts, seeds, dairy products, and fortified products.

Top 10 Healing Antioxidants

Antioxidants may play a key role in protecting your body against wear and tear and helping to reduce inflammation. The U.S. Department of Agriculture ranks the following fruits and vegetables according to their ability to act as antioxidants. From highest to lowest, they are:

1. Blueberries
2. Kale
3. Strawberries
4. Spinach
5. Brussels sprouts
6. Plums
7. Broccoli
8. Beetroot
9. Oranges
10. Red grapes

Food Sources of Pain-Free Minerals

Mineral	Food Source
Boron	Onions, garlic
Calcium	Dairy, tofu, dark green vegetables, sardines with bones
Copper	Shellfish, asparagus, nuts, whole grains, apples
Fluorine	Spinach, peas, beetroot, whole grains, sweet potatoes
Iodine	Seafood, seaweed, iodized salt
Magnesium	Tomatoes, mushrooms, cucumbers, potatoes, green vegetables
Manganese	Avocados, unrefined cereals, dark bread, tea, ginger, nuts, seeds, turnip greens
Phosphorus	Seeds, nuts, legumes, grains
Potassium	Vegetables, cabbage, spinach, bananas, fruit, bran flakes
Selenium	Cereals, garlic, nuts, seafood, wheat, soy
Zinc	Whole grains, oysters, nuts, seeds, green leafy vegetables

The Pain-Free Arthritis Diet

Until recently it's been unclear whether changing your diet may influence the symptoms of a chronic illness like arthritis. Nevertheless, new research continues to pour in touting the healing benefits of certain foods. Perhaps these foods aren't the miracle cure many hoped for, but through scientific studies we do know that certain nutrients can boost immune function and decrease inflammation in those with arthritis. Be sure to include the following suggestions in your pain-free diet to further reduce inflammation and pain.

Sip Tea

You can now add tea to your list of healing foods. In fact, some experts claim that we should add tea to the list of disease-fighting fruits and vegetables that we should eat daily. Some intriguing information was presented at the Society of Critical Care Medicine in January 2002 on how green tea may help decrease inflammation.

Green tea contains a type of polyphenol known as epigallocatechin-3-gallate, or EGCG, that inhibits the expression of the interleukin-8 gene. This is a key gene involved in the arthritis-inflammatory response. In these findings, researchers theorized that "more may be better" when it comes to green tea reducing the inflammatory response as EGCG short-circuits the process that leads to inflammation. (If you like black tea, drink up! Black tea is made from the same leaves as green and contains theaflavins, strong phytochemicals that help to protect the body. Though processed differently, black tea may be equally effective and is tolerable for many people.)

Sipping tea instead of other drinks may help to ward off painful fractures. In another revealing study published in May 2002 in the journal *Archives of Internal Medicine*, scientists found that men and women who drank tea for years had denser bones at three different skeletal sites, regardless of the type or amount of tea they consumed each day. Researchers concluded that drinking tea regularly for at least ten years was estimated to boost bone mineral density by up to 5 percent. This bone-boosting benefit may be attributed to special compounds in tea such as fluoride, phytoestrogens, and flavonoids, a group of antioxidants all working together. (Herbal teas are not "real" tea.) Some key prevention benefits of tea includes the following:

- Antioxidant
- Antibacterial
- Antivirus
- Antiaging
- Anti-inflammatory

Snack on Grapes

Resveratrol, a phytoestrogen, or plant-derived, nonsteroidal compound, is present in the skins of grapes, in mulberries, nuts, wine, and other foods. While all wines have some resveratrol, red wine seems to be the best source.

In the past few years, various studies have shown that resveratrol blocks cell inflammation, which is linked to arthritis and other diseases. A team of researchers now concludes that trans-resveratrol blocks the activation of the gene identified as COX-2, which is important in creating the inflammation that causes arthritis pain. This natural food substance is the first compound identified that both blocks the COX-2 gene from being activated and inactivates the enzyme created by that gene. Some believe that trans-resveratrol may turn out to be an improvement on aspirin in fighting diseases associated with COX-2, such as arthritis. For now, snack on grapes. They are low in fat and calories, and add some healing nutrients to your body.

Serve Vegetables

There is a lot of evidence that a diet high in vegetables can help to decrease inflammation in susceptible people. I've had many patients, particularly those with inflammatory types of arthritis, say a modified vegetarian diet (including fish) helps to reduce symptoms. Journal studies over the past five years have shown that a vegetarian diet causes an extensive change in the profile of the fatty acids of the serum phospholipids. These changes may favor production of prostaglandins and leukotrienes with less inflammatory activity, which is a bonus for those with inflammatory illnesses.

The vegetarian diet may also benefit those with inflammatory diseases because animal sources such as meat, poultry, dairy, and egg yolks contain arachidonic acid, a fatty acid that is converted to inflammatory prostaglandins and leukotrienes. Some holistic nutritionists believe that eliminating animal foods from the diet may significantly reduce inflammation and pain.

Boost Broccoli

Broccoli contains glutathione, a powerful antioxidant and detoxifying agent. In fact, without glutathione, other antioxidants such as vitamins C and E cannot do their job and protect you adequately against disease. Some new findings indicate that people who are low in this antioxidant are more likely to have arthritis than those who have higher amounts. Other glutathione-rich foods include asparagus, cabbage, cauliflower, potatoes, and tomatoes. Fruits with glutathione include avocados, grapefruit, oranges, peaches, and watermelon.

Feast on Fish

Studies continue to come in touting the benefits of omega-3 fatty acids, contained in fish, as helping to decrease inflammation. In a study published in May 1996 in the journal *Epidemiology*, scientists found that women who ate two or more servings of broiled or baked fish a week had about half the risk of getting rheumatoid arthritis as women who ate only one serving. Researchers estimate women with the best odds against RA were averaging a minimum 1.6 grams of omega-3 fatty acids daily, or the equivalent of 5 ounces or 140g of cooked rainbow trout.

Some research indicates that when fish oils are added to the diet, scientists measure a very significant drop in one of the most inflammatory immune substances—leukotriene B4, which is an important part of the process of inflammation in many types of arthritis. Researchers suspect that omega-3s may block the production of inflammatory substances linked to autoimmune diseases like rheumatoid arthritis and lupus. In some trials, taking fish-oil supplements for at least twelve weeks resulted in positive improvements in symptoms with less morning stiffness and tender joints.

Another study, published in the January 2000 issue of the *American Journal of Clinical Nutrition*, confirmed the healing benefits of omega-3 fatty acids. Researchers concluded that patients with rheumatoid arthritis who took dietary supplements of omega-3 fatty acids (EPA or eicosahexacnoic acid) had fewer tender joints and morning stiffness. The effective dose may be between 3 to 5 grams of the acids daily, although regulated guidelines have not been established regarding supplements of fish oil.

Researchers at Cardiff University in Wales found that cod-liver oil—the fishy tonic people used to take for "what ails them"—is effective in treating arthritic joint pain and even slowing or reversing the destruction of joint cartilage. Again, the omega-3 fatty acids in the oil are credited for "switching off" the collagen-degrading enzymes that break down joint cartilage. This leads to a slower progression of cartilage destruction, and reduces inflammation and the subsequent pain.

Because of the mercury content in some fish, including shark, swordfish, and marlin, the Food Standards Agency (FSA) recommends that

Eat Fish High in Omega-3

Anchovies	Salmon
Kippers	Sardines
Pilchards	Shad
Dogfish	Sturgeon
Herring	Fresh tuna
Mackerel	Trout

Include More Omega-3s

To add even more omega-3s to your daily diet, use rapeseed or flaxseed oil in cooking or salad dressings. Take borage seed oil or evening primrose oil—both available at most health food stores in a variety of forms. These oils are high in the plant form of omega-3, alpha-linolenic fatty acid. Your body converts this fat to one of the omega-3s found in fish oil.

pregnant or nursing women avoid these fish and limit their intake of fresh and canned tuna.

Pick Pineapple

For years, professional coaches have recommended pineapple to athletes to help heal sports injuries. That's because a key enzyme in pineapple called bromelain helps reduce inflammation. This may benefit those with knee osteoarthritis and rheumatoid arthritis, according to a German study that found bromelain enzymes resulted in a statistical reduction of pain. For those with carpal tunnel syndrome, some findings show eating pineapple is associated with reduced tissue swelling.

Add Olive Oil

A Greek study published in 1999 in the *American Journal of Clinical Nutrition* reported that eating large quantities of olive oil and cooked vegetables over a lifetime might cut the risk of developing rheumatoid arthritis. Researchers were unsure how olive oil reduces the risk for this inflammatory arthritis, but theorized that it may be due to its high concentrations of unsaturated fatty acids. One in particular, oleic acid, forms chemicals in the body that can decrease inflammation.

Another interesting point researchers made in this study is that raw vegetables did not appear to give as much protection as cooked vegetables. This may be because the heat from cooking breaks down the plant cell walls and increases absorption of healing compounds that may help those with inflammatory arthritis.

Serve Soy

In some new findings presented in early 2002 at the American Pain Society, researchers at Johns Hopkins University in Baltimore concluded that a diet rich in soy that reduced pain and swelling in rats may one day be used by humans to manage chronic pain. In the study, scientists found that rats fed a soy-based diet experienced "significantly less" swelling and were able to tolerate more pain than another test group given a milk protein. The pain tolerance was determined by assessing how long rats could endure pressure and heat stimulus before removing their paw from the heat supply. Of course, we have a long way to go before proving the same result in humans, but this study is positive.

Along with the possibility of decreasing pain, soy foods have other great benefits, including being dairy free, low in saturated fat, and excellent meat substitutes. For years, soybeans have played an integral part in the Asian culture with heart disease, breast cancer, prostate cancer, and osteoporosis rates much lower for Asian men and women than for Americans. In addition, isoflavones, phytochemicals found in soy, are close in structure to the body's form of estrogen. While these plant ingredients mimic the hormone estrogen, they appear to have no harmful side effects and may give a bonus in relieving menopausal symptoms

Soy Sources

Soy Food	Grams of Protein
Tofu	10 grams per ½ cup
Soy milk	7 grams per 1 cup
Soy yogurt	7 grams per 1 cup
Miso	2 grams per tablespoon
Black soybeans	9 grams per ½ cup
Green soybeans (edamame)	11 grams per ½ cup
Tempeh	16 grams per ½ cup
Textured soy protein	11 grams per ¼ cup
Soy nuts	22 grams per ½ cup

Eat Ample Protein

Eat 1 to 1.2 grams of protein per kilogram of body weight (to make up for the protein lost in the inflammatory process).

Include Healing Foods

Broccoli	Pineapple
Grapes	Soy
Tea (green or black)	Vegetables
Fish	

Increase Flavonoid-Rich Foods

Flavonoids are a family of more than four thousand compounds that include polyphenols and give color to fruits and vegetables. These nutrients are powerful antioxidants and may hold the key to disease prevention. Polyphenols act like antioxidants or rust-proofing agents, which are thought to reduce the cellular oxidation.

Although more studies are needed to claim these nutrients prevent inflammation or disease, try to include flavonoid-rich foods in your daily diet including green tea, onions, apples, soy, and grapes, among others.

---

and helping to prevent osteoporosis. In a study published in the January 2001 issue of *Obstetrics and Gynecology*, researchers suggested that a diet rich in soy might help women retain strong bones and reduce the risk of painful and debilitating fractures.

Try the Pain-Free Food Elimination Diet

Many doctors believe that a type of allergic immune-system reaction to foods may occur in some patients' joints. Still, it's hard to know if and how a certain food triggers arthritis symptoms. Many patients claim that avoiding certain foods helps them to realize less pain. Others eliminate the same foods and receive no benefit at all—except for missing favorite foods they stopped eating!

Food allergy refers to an undesirable immunologic reaction to the protein in foods. Although researchers are still unsure about the arthritis-food allergy connection, we do know that asthma, allergies, rashes, and hives are examples of immune-system reactions, and sometimes food is the culprit. Identifying and eliminating the food protein from the diet may resolve the symptoms.

Some interesting findings supporting the food-pain link were reported in October 2001 at the annual meeting of the American College of Nutrition. Researchers suggested that people with fibromyalgia might experience reductions in symptoms if they eliminate one or more foods from their diet. In the study, the scientists reviewed medical histories of fibromyalgia patients who agreed to eliminate foods such as wheat, corn, dairy, citrus, soy, and nuts from their daily diet. After two weeks without eating any of these potential food allergens, nearly half of the patients reported a significant reduction of pain. Other symptoms such as heartburn, breathing difficulties, bloating, headache, and fatigue were also reduced. After the elimination phase ended, patients then began to introduce a specific food every two or three days and symptoms such as pain and headache began to return.

Some of my patients with inflammatory arthritis have found that certain foods trigger symptoms, particularly corn, dairy, wheat, soy products, citrus fruits, eggs, red meat, sugar, fats, salt, and caffeine, among others. Although the number is small, a few patients find that by eliminating the nightshade plants (tomatoes, white potatoes, all peppers, and eggplant), they are able to experience symptom relief. The nightshade plants are thought to increase symptoms because of a substance called solanine, which could be toxic if not destroyed in the intestine and might lead to the worsening of arthritis symptoms. Of course, some foods can trigger gouty arthritis, especially with those people who have difficulty processing chemicals that are in coffee, organ meats, herring, sardines, scallops, and anchovies. Eliminating these foods and giving up alcohol— another gout trigger—can greatly reduce the painful attacks.

Phase I: Elimination
Eliminate the following foods for two weeks:

1. Corn (popcorn, corn chips, corn syrups, corn starches, and by-products)
2. Dairy (milk, butter, ice cream, yogurt, cheese, and other by-products)
3. Wheat (all breads, crackers, biscuits, noodles, and other by-products)
4. Citrus (oranges, grapefruits, lemons, limes, and other citrus and juices)
5. Tomato (pizza, spaghetti sauce, ketchup, and tomato by-products)
6. Yeast (dried fruits, vinegar, mushrooms, bread, pickles, and beer)

7. Soybean (soy sauce, soy lecithin, and tofu)
8. Carob (egg, chocolate, colas, beans, peas, peanuts, and peanut butter)

Be sure that the remaining foods in your diet during the Elimination Phase supply you with adequate nutrition, and supplement with a multivitamin. Foods that are allowed during the elimination process include many fresh meats, poultry, fish, vegetables, and fruits (except the listed varieties), rice, cereals, and water.

A Patient's Food Elimination Diary

Trial and error is an age-old scientific principle. For those with arthritis, sometimes trial and error can pay off as you find what helps your pain and stiffness—and what causes it to worsen. After following the Pain-Free Food Elimination Diet, forty-five-year-old Ben, a corporate executive with rheumatoid arthritis, realized that certain foods increased his pain and stiffness. Here is what he wrote in his Pain-Free Diary:

> I had reason to question food triggers for my rheumatoid arthritis. In the past, I'd had reactions to monosodium glutamate, shellfish, and additives in fast-food milkshakes that caused blinding headaches. When I ate at restaurants, I often could not sleep that night because of increased pain and inflammation. So, I decided to modify my healthy diet to exclude "stressor" foods such as caffeine, chocolate, peanut butter, nuts, and alcohol. In my modified diet, I increased raw vegetables, fruits, brown rice, fresh fish (salmon, tuna, trout), beans, gluten and wheat-free bread, and green tea.
>
> Over a period of weeks, I began to experiment with foods to see if I reacted to them. For instance, cashews and mixed nuts seem to cause an increase in inflammation and pain in the hands within two hours of eating. I also reacted to a can of organic tomato soup with increased inflammation in the hands.
>
> I am convinced that elimination of certain foods, along with increasing raw fruits and vegetables, has helped to decrease my pain and inflammation. I have reduced my pain medication from four pills per day to three, and the need for medication now extends to every six hours instead of every four hours. In the first two weeks of my new diet, I reduced my prednisone from 14 milligrams daily to 10 milligrams.
>
> I don't believe my diet will "cure" me from rheumatoid arthritis. However, eliminating certain foods and adding healing nutrients has given me more control of my chronic illness and lets me decrease the dependency on pain medications. In my case, RA flares were triggered by food reactions. I now feel in control that I can reduce the number of flares.flares were triggered by food reactions. I now feel in control that I can reduce the number of flares.

Phase II: Reintroduction

After a period of strict abstinence from the listed foods, reintroduce the foods, one at a time. Take only a small amount of the food initially to see if there is any reaction. If there is no reaction, then eat more of this food in larger amounts. Also, try by-products of the food to see if these are well tolerated. If there is no change in arthritis symptoms, go to the next category and reintroduce this food. If you notice symptoms, stop the newly introduced food until the symptoms clear, and move on to the next food category.

Use the Food Elimination Diet chart (below) to keep a record of the foods you reintroduce and any symptoms you feel after eating. If you believe the food worsens your symptoms, talk to your doctor or a registered dietitian to see how to make healthy changes in your diet.

Food Elimination Diet

	What I Ate	How I Felt: 30 minutes	How I Felt: 1 hour	How I Felt: 2–3 hours	How I Felt: 12 hours
Breakfast					
Snack					
Lunch					
Snack					
Dinner					
Snack					

Avoid the Pain-Boosters

Just as researchers are discovering healing foods, other foods may increase inflammation and pain. Just as with the Pain-Free Food Elimination Diet, the only way you'll know if these foods influence your arthritis symptoms is to eliminate them for at least two weeks, then slowly reintroduce them into your diet.

Avoid Omega-6 Fatty Acids

Linoleic or omega-6 fatty acids, a type of unsaturated fat in corn and safflower oil, may do the opposite of the healing omega-3s in the body. A revealing study published in the December 1999 issue of the *American Journal of Clinical Nutrition* indicates that omega-6 fatty acids might activate genes that promote inflammation and reduce the cells' ability to protect themselves from oxidative damage caused by free radicals that can damage body tissues. Considering the escalating number of auto-immune diseases that are at epidemic proportions in a society that thrives on junk food (high in omega-6 fatty acids), this study is highly revealing.

Avoid Decaffeinated Coffee

There is also new information from the Iowa Women's Health Study targeting decaffeinated coffee as increasing a woman's risk of developing rheumatoid arthritis. In the study, researchers found that those who drank caffeinated coffee were not at increased risk, while those who drank three or more cups of tea *reduced their risk* of rheumatoid arthritis by 60 percent.

Watch Your Grains

Another interesting study, published in the April 2000 issue of the *British Journal of Nutrition*, suggests that eating cereal grains may promote the development of rheumatoid arthritis. Researchers state that cereal grains have a substance known as lectins, which can come into the body from the digestive tract, prompting an immune response. These scientists speculate that this may eventually lead to an immune system attack on the joints. Although this finding is theory right now, it does show you how much we are learning about the human body and its response to the foods we eat.

How Medications Interfere

- Cause a poor or uncontrollable appetite
- Enhance or hinder the body's absorption of vitamins and minerals and other nutrients
- Change the way the body uses vitamins, minerals, and other nutrients
- Change the rate at which the body gets rid of vitamins, minerals, and other nutrients

---

Food-Medication Interaction

Medication plays a vital role in the management of arthritis. However, serious problems can result when medicine is not taken as directed. Reactions to a medication can often seem worse than the pain it is intended to treat. For example, many patients find that nonsteroidal anti-inflammatory drugs cause stomach irritation. Aspirin may cause reflux of stomach acid in the esophagus, resulting in heartburn.

Be Aware of Interactions

By being aware of possible food-drug interactions that occur with your medications, you can minimize the adverse effects. Food can influence the absorption of your medication, so it is wise to know how a medication should be taken. Whether your stomach is full or empty can decrease, delay, or even increase the absorption of your medication. Certain drugs should be taken on an empty stomach to enhance absorption into the bloodstream, such as thyroid replacement medications. Other drugs should be taken with food in the stomach in order to prevent irritation or stomach upset, such as the traditional nonsteroid anti-inflammatory drugs (page 159) or oral cortisone derivatives such as prednisone or other corticosteroids. The new NSAIDs (COX 1135) can be taken with or without food.

Doctor's Pain-Free Treatment

Can the nutrition plan help you? Even if you are currently eating a balanced diet, review the information in this step and see if changing your diet, along with healthy weight loss, may help you achieve a pain-free life.

Let's Review: 8 Steps to Getting Started with the Pain-Free Nutrition Plan

1. Talk to your doctor about your normal diet and weight-loss needs, if any. Ask if there are any restrictions to making dietary changes.
2. Set a target weight and then calculate the number of calories needed daily to reach that target (see page 35). Divide the number of calories by six to give you the average number of calories available for mini-meals.
3. If you need to lose weight, review the Glycemic Index information (page 37) and plan to choose foods at the lowest end of this chart. These foods will help you to eat less and keep your blood sugar level even.
4. Assess your average serving size, using the listings starting on page 38, and make adjustments to downsize any servings that are larger than normal.
5. Focus on whole foods, and make sure you get plenty of the healing vitamins and minerals discussed in this chapter, beginning on page 42.
6. Using the Pain-Free Food Elimination Diet, keep accurate accounts of any foods that cause increased pain or other symptoms. Be sure to report this change to your doctor for evaluation.
7. Add fish at least three times a week to boost omega-3 fatty acids, a proven aid in reducing inflammation. Consider the other healing foods such as soy or tea that are proven to decrease inflammation.
8. Notice any reactions you might have to medications when taken with or without food and talk to your doctor about changes that might be made.

Osteoarthritis

- Set weight-loss goals and follow the strategies for reducing calories and using the glycemic index. Keep a Pain-Free Diary to make sure you are following the suggestions accurately.
- Review the vitamins and minerals in this step. Make sure you eat foods in each category to supply these needs; add supplements, if your diet lacks in these nutrients.
- Try the Pain-Free Food Elimination Diet.
- Consider avoiding animal foods including meat, poultry, eggs, and dairy products to see if your pain is reduced.

- Avoid nightshade plants (tomatoes, white potatoes, all peppers, and eggplant) to see if you get symptom relief.
- Include healing foods such as broccoli, grapes, tea (green or black, not decaffeinated), fish, pineapple, soy, and plenty of fresh vegetables.

Fibromyalgia

- Make sure you are at a healthy weight. If you need to lose weight, use foods low on the Glycemic Index.
- Use mini-meals to help keep your energy level up and your blood sugar level steady.
- Increase fresh fruits and vegetables in your diet. Focus on vegetables high in magnesium, such as bananas and tofu, which may help to reduce pain. Select fruits and vegetables high in vitamin C to ensure immune function and to boost concentration.
- Try the Pain-Free Food Elimination Diet to see if specific foods influence the pain you feel.
- Include healing foods such as broccoli, grapes, tea (green or black, not decaffeinated), fish, pineapple, soy, and plenty of fresh vegetables.

Carpal Tunnel Syndrome

- Make sure you don't have a vitamin B_6 deficiency. Eating whole foods is the best way to ensure adequate absorption of nutrients. Fortified cereal has up to 100 percent of the RDA of vitamin B_6, and one banana plus one half-cup or 80g of chickpeas gives you more than the RDA of vitamin B_6.

Bursitis and Tendonitis

- Make sure your daily diet is well balanced and filled with the pain-free foods that are high in antioxidants, vitamins, and minerals.
- Be sure to focus on a diet filled with fresh fruits and vegetables and reduce your intake of animal protein to help ease inflammation.

Rheumatoid Arthritis (and Other Inflammatory Arthritis)

- Focus on the foods listed on page 57 to help decrease inflammation; use the Pain-Free Food Elimination Diet, page 57, to see which foods may aggravate your condition.
- If you take corticosteroids, this may block calcium absorption and result in bone loss. Make sure you have adequate calcium and

vitamin D in your diet or supplement (see pages 45 and 48 for recommended dosage).

• If you take the disease-modifying anti-rheumatic drug methotrexate, be sure you also take a multivitamin/mineral supplement that has 400 micrograms of folic acid.

• Review the foods high in vitamin E and make sure to include plenty of these in your daily diet, along with the other foods in this step.

• Be sure to eat fatty fish several times each week to boost omega-3 fatty acids in the body.

• Avoid decaffeinated beverages.

• Experiment eliminating various nightshade plants (tomatoes, white potatoes, all peppers, and eggplant) and try the Pain-Free Food Elimination Diet to see if you get symptom relief.

• Include healing foods such as broccoli, grapes, tea (green or black, not decaffeinated), fish, pineapple, soy, and plenty of fresh vegetables.

Gout

• Avoid foods containing purines, chemicals found in coffee, organ meats, herring, sardines, scallops, and anchovies.

• Avoid alcohol in large amounts.

Try Alternative Therapies

If you suffer from the side effects of some arthritis medications, including stomach distress, fatigue, or weight gain, I'm sure you've considered natural therapies for pain relief. Mark, a forty-seven-year-old clinical psychologist, knows all about arthritis pain and the side effects of harsh medications. After all, he has lived with the pain of osteoarthritis since he injured his knee in a motorcycle accident more than a decade ago. Although nonsteroid anti-inflammatory drugs (NSAIDs) helped to end the pain for a while, Mark disliked the medication, saying it made him "feel drowsy and foggy." The medications also upset his stomach, causing frequent heartburn and gastrointestinal problems.

Mark started taking the natural dietary supplement glucosamine, a joint-maintenance supplement made from shellfish. He continued taking NSAIDs and doing twice-daily moist heat soaks and regular exercise, including riding his stationary bike, to keep the knee joint flexible and the muscles strong. After two weeks of taking glucosamine, Mark reported a dramatic reduction in pain and stiffness during exercise. Within two months, he stopped taking the NSAID and is virtually pain-free today.

I cannot promise that every arthritis patient who takes glucosamine will have dramatic results like Mark. However, I do know that some natural supplements can safely complement your Pain-Free Program and sometimes let you reduce medications.

Understanding the Causes of Pain

In the first two steps of your Pain-Free Program, you discovered why exercise is the gold standard treatment for ending arthritis pain and stiffness. You also learned that decreasing your weight may decrease your pain, and adding certain foods may give you another healing boost by reducing inflammation. Before I explain some safe alternative therapies in this step, it's important to understand the substances in the body that cause pain, including prostaglandins, cytokines, and peptides such as Substance P, among others.

Prostaglandins are the chemicals that cause inflammation, pain, and swelling and even joint destruction in some types of inflammatory arthritis. *Substance P*, a neuropeptide in the brain, is also involved in pain signals. This chemical helps nervous system cells send messages to one another about painful stimuli. It is thought that when Substance P levels are elevated in the body, they may produce higher levels of pain.

Cytokines are proteins that carry messages between cells and regulate immunity and inflammation. Two cytokines, TNF (tumor necrosis factor) and IL-1 (interleukin one), play essential roles in the cartilage destruction and inflammation process. *Tumor necrosis factor*, a protein made of amino acids, is an important product of the cells that create inflammation. In rheumatoid arthritis, TNF is overproduced in the joints. Researchers believe that TNF causes inflammation, resulting in destruction of bone and cartilage. TNF can also cause pain, fever, weight loss, and the fatigue associated with rheumatoid arthritis. Understanding that TNF may trigger many other enzymes, scientists now believe that blocking TNF can greatly relieve the effects of inflammation.

While exciting new medications have been developed to block chemicals such as prostaglandins or TNF, experts believe that herbs and other alternative therapies may have an effect in arthritis. For instance, the over-the-counter supplement quercetin is a highly concentrated form of bioflavonoids, naturally found in citrus fruits, red and yellow onions, and broccoli. Some studies indicate that quercetin may benefit those with gout (a form of arthritris) because it inhibits uric acid production in a similar way as the pharmaceutical allopurinol. Quercetin also inhibits the release of prostaglandins, blocking these inflammatory compounds from causing swelling and pain.

Other studies confirm that patients with rheumatoid arthritis may benefit from supplements of selenium, which reduce the production of

---

Gather Your Pain-Free Tools

1. Use your Pain-Free Diary to record any natural therapies you try, including the name, dosage, and side effects, if any.
2. Be sure to talk with your doctor before taking any medication or natural dietary supplement. Also, talk with your doctor about drug-supplement interaction and any side effects after taking herbs or other supplements.

---

inflammatory prostaglandins and leukotrienes. Cat's claw, a common herbal remedy for pain, is often recommended as an "immune stimulator." It is thought that cat's claw may inhibit inflammatory cytokines in cases of chronic inflammation.

Natural Therapies Help Resolve Pain

I often recommend natural therapies to help resolve pain. Some of these herbs or nutrients inhibit the system's inflammatory cytokines, which otherwise would become elevated in chronic pain conditions. Others block the pain-causing prostaglandins and leukotrienes that cause inflammation. Some of the therapies boost endorphins, the body's natural opioids that relieve pain; others help heal an exhausted immune system and repair damaged tissue.

As I've learned more about natural therapies, I realize that they may just emerge as the best strategies, especially for those with mild to moderate arthritis pain. I understand that a great deal of uncertainty

---

Red Flag!

Sometimes a supplement or herb may counteract the effects of your prescription medication, leaving your doctor baffled when the medicine is ineffective and your arthritis worse. A natural therapy may cause liver damage or other serious side effects. That's why I always remind my patients to use caution with any unproven treatment. As a rule of thumb, just because something is natural does not mean that it is always safe. As Socrates realized, hemlock, a poisonous plant, is very natural—but it is also deadly!

---

surrounds these alternative therapies because they have not been tested as rigorously as medications, but this does not mean they do not work. (A lot of medications used daily have been tested and still have serious or even deadly side effects.) I've found that some natural therapies may work well for one patient, yet do nothing for another patient. In addition, most alternative treatments work best in conjunction with prescribed medical therapies. That's why talking openly with your doctor before you take any unproven treatment will help you get the best of both worlds and find the safest treatments that work for you.

Dietary Supplements

A decade ago, the most popular dietary supplement was a vitamin-mineral supplement. Herbal ingredients were scarce, and most people hadn't heard of glucosamine, the popular arthritis pain-relieving supplement made from shrimp, crab, and lobster shells. Today in the United States, dietary supplements include a wide assortment of products, including multivitamins, minerals, amino acids, herbs, as well as ingredients derived from plant and animal sources. These are available in an assortment of forms, from capsules, pills, and gel tabs to liquids, tinctures, extracts, and powders.

While the dietary supplement industry is not regulated by the Food and Drug Administration (FDA), in 1994 the FDA established standards for manufacturers assuring that supplements bear ingredient and nutritional labeling. For instance, according to the FDA, herbal supplements must state the part of the plant from which the ingredient is derived. A herbal supplement such as black cohosh, commonly taken by women to decrease symptoms of menopause, might state on the label "Black Cohosh extract (root) containing 2.5 percent Triterpene Glycosides . . . 160 mg. Other ingredients: Rice Powder, Silicon Dioxide, Magnesium Stearate, Gelatin." Other than that, manufacturers are free to make whatever claims they want on the supplement label or in literature, and there is no assurance that these claims are valid.

That's why you need to be cautious when choosing dietary supplements, including herbal remedies. I have no doubt that some herbal treatments are highly effective for easing pain or helping other symptoms subside. In fact, I take several dietary supplements each morning before I attend to patients at the clinics. Nevertheless, I am also selective when it comes to the type of supplement and the manufacturing brand.

Herbal Remedies to Ease Pain

While most medications today are synthetic, composed of laboratory-made chemicals, about 80 percent of the medicines listed in the British Pharmacopoeia, the authoritative collection of standards for medicines in the United Kingdom for almost 140 years, were plant-based at some time, such as aspirin. Herbal therapies work by directly interacting with the body chemistry. Some herbs are ingested through the mouth and into the bloodstream via the digestive system. Others are rubbed on the skin and then move into the bloodstream.

When choosing herbs, look for those labeled "standardized." This means the manufacturer measured the amount of key ingredients in the herbal batch. Since plants can vary greatly in their potency and there is no government regulation for ingredients in herbal remedies, the chances are better that you will get what you pay for in a "standardized brand." Also buy herbs from a reputable manufacturer instead of an off-brand that may be cheaper. Some of the known brands I prefer include General Nutrition, Natrol, Sundown, Your Life, Mother Nature, and Nature's Bounty. Not all of these brands are avaliable in the UK, but they can all be ordered online.

Don't forget that dosing is not exact with dietary supplements or herbs, and the potency can vary. That's why you must do your homework before taking the latest herbal "cure." I have given you recommended doses in Step 3 after compiling data from the *Physician's Desk Reference for Herbal Therapies* and Germany's Commission E (similar to our FDA) and having it confirmed by the American Botanical Council. With your physician's permission, start with that dose and stay on it for two weeks. Most patients find the suggested "serving size" is adequate in giving them relief.

Herbs vary in price depending on where they are purchased, how they are processed, and the strength of the herb. You may find that when herbs are calibrated so the active ingredient is measured exactly, they are also more expensive. Some of the more expensive brands, such as Nature's Answer, calibrate their herbs and use only organic products. Sometimes these supplements may provide more of the healing element you are trying to ingest. If the herb is not calibrated, it may provide too little—or even too much of the active ingredient.

For instance, ingesting too much salicin, the active ingredient in white willow bark, may cause gastrointestinal problems as it is gradually converted to salicylic acid in the intestine and liver. Aspirin (acetylsalicylic

---

Commonly Used Herbal Preparations

- Oils: Extracted essential plant oils that are combined with a vegetable oil for massage or aromatherapy.
- Tinctures: Herb essences that are steeped in alcohol solution.
- Capsules: Gelatin containers filled with lightly powdered herbs, oils, or extracted juice.
- Liniments: Extracts of herbs in an oil or spirit base that is applied to the skin.
- Poultices: Gauze or linen wrapped around herbal therapy and then applied directly to skin.

---

acid), a synthetic replacement for salicin, can also cause stomach upset and ulcers. But getting the right amount of white willow bark can help to decrease inflammation and pain without all of the aspirin side effects. In this case, having your herb calibrated to ensure the proper amount may be helpful in the end.

Miraculous as these remedies may seem, always talk to a health care professional before taking any nonstandard therapy or natural dietary supplement. If you decide to take the following herbal supplements, play it safe and talk to your doctor, pharmacist, or a certified nutritionist about side effects. Herbal therapies are not recommended for pregnant women, children, the elderly, or those with compromised immune systems.

Herbs to Reduce Pain

Boswellia (*Boswellia serrata*), the gummy resin of the boswellia tree, has a long history of use as an anti-inflammatory. This herb inhibits leukotrienes and other pro-inflammatory mediators in the body and improves the blood supply to joint tissues. Boswellic acids are thought to suppress the proliferating tissue found in the inflamed areas and also put a stop to the breakdown of connective tissue.

How to use: Use in tincture, dried leaves and stems, or capsules. Unlike nonsteroidal anti-inflammatory drugs (NSAIDs), boswellia does not cause stomach upset.

Cat's claw (*Uncaria tomentosa*), a powerful botanical, comes from the Amazon Peruvian rain forest. With its anti-inflammatory and anti-rheumatic properties, cat's claw is often used for treating arthritis and fibromyalgia. This herb also has a rich source of pycnogenol, a powerful antioxidant and free radical scavenger (see Vitamin E, page 46) that boosts immune function. Cat's claw has alkaloids and other constituents that account for the anti-inflammatory and antioxidant actions.

How to use: Take in dried or powdered form compressed into capsules.

Devil's claw (*Harpagophytum procumbens*), a bitter herb, has properties similar to the nonsteroid anti-inflammatory drugs and is commonly used to treat arthritis, back pain, and rheumatic pains. This herb is widely used in Europe as a treatment for arthritis pain.

How to use: Take in tablet form, as it's extremely bitter in teas.

Evening primrose (*Oenothera biennis*), a sweet herb, is used to treat inflammatory conditions and has been recommended for arthritis because the oil contains gamma-linolenic acid (GLA)—also found in borage seeds and blackcurrant seeds. GLA is an essential fatty acid (EFA) that helps to reduce inflammation associated with allergic response by aiding in the production of prostaglandins that counter inflammation.

How to use: Take in capsule form.

Feverfew (*Tanacetum parthenium L*) reduces inflammation as well as prostaglandins. This common herb contains a variety of compounds known as sesquiterpene lactones. More than 85 percent of these are a compound called parthenolide, which is said to inhibit the release of serotonin and some inflammatory mediators. Feverfew's actions might resemble those of aspirin, and it may help to reduce pain.

How to use: Take the dried plant compressed in tablets or capsules to inhibit inflammation. Or make feverfew tea by steeping one teaspoon of dried plant in two cups of water for 15 minutes. Caution: Anyone with a clotting disorder should consult a physician before taking feverfew. Do not take feverfew with a nonsteroidal anti-inflammatory drug, aspirin, or warfarin because it can increase the chance of bleeding.

Ginger (*Zingiber officinale*), used for centuries in Traditional Chinese Medicine and the Ayurvedic system of medicine, has been shown to reduce inflammation and symptoms of osteoarthritis in clinical studies. In some new research published in the November 2001 issue of *Arthritis and Rheumatism*, 63 percent of the patients with osteoarthritis of the knee who took ginger reported reduced pain in the knee while standing and less pain after walking 50 feet. Although there were no serious side effects with the ginger extract, some volunteers in the study reported gastrointestinal discomfort such as heartburn and burping. Studies are being done at some medical centers on using ginger externally to ease arthritis pain.

How to use: Use in tincture, dried leaves and stems, capsules, or in spice on foods. Also, boil ginger root for a soothing tea.

Myrrh (*Commiphora myrrha*), a bitter and spicy herb with anti-spasmodic properties, is used to treat arthritis and rheumatic pain and can be combined with goldenseal or garlic to be used for most acute anti-inflammatory conditions.

How to use: Take as capsules for a short period (one or two weeks). Do not use if you are pregnant.

Nettle (*Urtica urens*), a bland and bitter herb with properties that counteract inflammation, contains a variety of natural chemicals that may help to lower pain and swelling. These chemicals also help slow down the actions of many enzymes that trigger inflammation, such as cyclooxygen-ase and lipooxygenase. Nettle leaf has been used for years in Germany as a safe treatment of arthritis. In a study published in the May 2000 issue of the *Journal of the Royal Society of Medicine*, researchers at the University of Plymouth applied stinging nettle leaves to the hands of twenty-seven arthritis sufferers. After one week, they found that stinging nettles not only significantly reduced pain, but that the level of pain stayed lower through most of the treatment. They concluded that nettles contain both serotonin and histamine, both of which are neurotransmitters, and might affect pain perception and transmission at the nerve endings. It is also thought that the nettle sting has an effect similar to acupuncture, or that it might have a counter irritant effect like capsaicin (see page 6).

How to use: Use tincture, dried leaves and stems, or capsules. *Caution:* Excessive amounts may cause stomach irritation, constipation, or burning skin. If you are allergic to pollen, avoid nettle.

Turmeric (*Curcuma longa*), a spicy and bitter herb with analgesic properties, is a member of the ginger family and a native of South Asia (probably India). Turmeric has a potent anti-inflammatory compound, curcumin, which protects the body against the ravages of free radicals, naturally occurring toxic substances.

How to use: Use as spice on foods, mixed in hot tea or warm milk, or in capsules.

White willow bark (*Salix alba*), a bitter herb with analgesic properties, has been called the first nonsteroid anti-inflammatory drug and has been used in ancient China as far back as 500 B.C. In a study published in the *British Journal of Rheumatology*, researchers compared

---

Red Alert!

While the Food and Drug Administration does not hold dietary supplements, including herbal treatments, to a pre-approval process as it does pharmaceuticals, the Dietary Supplement Health and Education Act of 1994 allows the FDA to remove a supplement or herbal therapy from the market if it appears that the product is not safe. The following herbs are considered too dangerous to use:

• *Yohimbe* is marketed worldwide as a male aphrodisiac and cure for impotence. It can cause panic attacks, as well as neurological and psychological effects and even death.

• *Chaparral* is from an American Southwest desert bush called creosote touted for its anti-aging properties, but known for causing terminal liver failure.

• *Ma huang* is one of several names for products containing ephedra. Common names for these evergreen plants include Mormon tea and squaw tea. Adverse effects include high blood pressure, nerve damage, rapid heart rate, stroke, and memory loss. Ma huang is found in both over-the-counter and prescription drugs, as well as in some weight-control products.

---

the effectiveness of willow bark (assalix) with a COX-2 inhibitor, a new "super" aspirin medication commonly used to treat arthritis pain. Both groups reported a decrease in pain. Researchers concluded that there was no significant difference in effectiveness between the two treatments at the doses chosen, but treatment with white willow bark was about 40 percent less expensive.

How to use: Soak one to three teaspoons of powdered bark (available at most health food stores) in cold water for two to five hours; take one-third cup three times daily. Caution: If you are allergic to aspirin and/or other NSAIDs, avoid taking willow bark. Also, you cannot take willow bark while taking any other traditional NSAID, including aspirin, ibuprofen, and others.

Herbs to Induce Relaxation and Sleep

If you have difficulty sleeping because of arthritis pain and stiffness, one of the following sleepy-time herbs might help to increase relaxation and calmness:

Chamomile (*Matricaria recutita*) depresses the central nervous system and may help relieve arthritic joint inflammation. This commonly used herb helps to calm anxiety and increase deep sleep. German chamomile is best used as a tea; Roman chamomile has a bitter taste and is more appropriate as a tincture. Both can be taken in tea or capsules to soothe nerves and induce sleepiness.

Passionflower (*Passiflora incarnata*) is used as a sedative in Europe and is generally ingested as a tea before bedtime. Passionflower is available in the form of teas, tinctures, capsules, and extracts. Take near bedtime for a restful night's sleep.

Valerian (*Valeriana officinalis*) is a spicy, bitter herb with sedative properties used to calm the central nervous system, making it useful for treating anxiety, insomnia, and stress. Take valerian in tea, tincture, or capsules about thirty minutes before bedtime to fall asleep easily.

Herbal Rubs

Some herbs work best to relieve pain when they are rubbed directly into the painful joint or muscle. Most herbal rubs, liniments, and poultices are called counter-irritants, meaning they work by pitting pain against pain, helping to stimulate the body to lower its pain sensitivity. Sometimes these rubs will cause local swelling or irritation when applied to the skin, causing the temperature of the skin to feel warm to the touch. This local reaction can result in a reduction of pain as the brain becomes over-whelmed with a new influx of chemical messages and becomes distract-ed from recognizing the pain source. Herbal rubs are highly effective and are available at most health food stores and drugstores.

Arnica (*Arnica montana*) has as active components *sesquiterpene lac-tones*, which are known to reduce inflammation and decrease pain. In ointment form, arnical tincture acts as an anti-inflammatory and anal-gesic for aches and bruises. *Caution:* If you have allergies, arnica may cause a skin rash in some people. Arnica should not be taken internally, as it can increase blood pressure and may damage the heart muscle.

Camphor (*Cinnamomum camphora*) is a gum resin extracted from leaves of the gum or laurel camphor tree. When used as an analgesic liniment, it can bring ample relief to the aches and pains of arthritis or fibromyalgia. Camphor is a key ingredient in many over-the-counter pain ointments.

Capsicum (*Capsicum frutesens*), a counter-irritant ointment made from the spice in cayenne pepper, is an effective treatment for muscle

Making Herbal Tea

Take 2 teaspoons of dried herbs per cup of boiling water. Put in a teapot or pot. Pour the boiling water on the herbs and cover. Let this brew for about 3 to 4 minutes, and then strain into a cup. Store the remaining tea in a tightly covered container in the refrigerator. Herbal tea lasts about three days in the refrigerator.

spasms and arthritis and to relieve pain caused by shingles and surgical scars. *Capsaicin*, the active ingredient in capsicum, temporarily stimulates the release of various neurotransmitters from the nerves, leading to their depletion. Without the neurotransmitters, pain signals can no longer be sent and arthritis patients get much-needed relief. While the cream causes a burning sensation the first few times, this should go away with each application. Wash your hands well after use to avoid getting in your eyes, nose, or mouth. If the cream is too irritating, discontinue usage.

Natural Supplements May Boost Healing

A host of dietary supplements show great promise in healing the ravaging pain of arthritis. While some got a bad rap a few years back, we now know that these supplements can and do alleviate pain if used correctly. Following are the supplements I recommend to patients.

Glucosamine

The over-the-counter natural supplement glucosamine works for many people to help lessen the pain and stiffness of arthritis. Glucosamine is a naturally occurring molecule in the body and plays an important role in the structure and repair of cartilage and other connective tissues. The supplement form of glucosamine comes from crab, lobster, and shrimp shells and has been found to help maintain lubrication in the joints, stimulate cartilage repair, and slow the breakdown of cartilage.

Some evidence published in the January 2001 issue of the *Lancet*, the British medical journal, confirmed that glucosamine might slow the progression of osteoarthritis. In the study, 212 people with osteoarthritis were randomly selected to receive either 1,500 milligrams of glucosamine each day or a placebo (a sugar pill). Researchers concluded that those patients who took glucosamine experienced less wear of the joint

---

Red Flag!

If you are allergic to shellfish or on a low iodine diet, avoid the glucosamine supplement. Or, if you are pregnant, do not take glucosamine since it has not been tested.

---

cartilage than those who took the placebo. This is especially good news for those who are aspirin sensitive or who cannot take NSAIDs because of allergy or gastrointestinal upset.

Because glucosamine is an unregulated dietary supplement, the quality of the product will vary, which means some brands may be ineffective for relief of pain. (The standard dose is 1,500 milligrams daily.)

Chondroitin

Chondroitin sulfate is another popular over-the-counter supplement that many of my patients use successfully to ease osteoarthritis symptoms. Some studies show that chondroitin reduces joint pain significantly and that overall mobility is significantly greater. Like glucosamine, chondroitin sulfate appears to be safe and effective for treating arthritis symptoms. There are no studies showing that both supplements are necessary for pain relief, even though manufacturers often mix the two supplements in over-the-counter pain formulas. (The standard dose is 1,200 milligrams daily of chondroitin.)

Melatonin

Almost all my patients complain about poor sleep, especially if their arthritis pain is uncontrolled. Prescription sleep aids may help for a while, but the side effects of daytime sleepiness and inattentiveness make

---

Copper Bracelets

Copper bracelets are commonly used by arthritis sufferers. It is their hope that the copper is in some way absorbed by the body to have a beneficial effect on arthritis. One survey found up to 45 percent of patients had used a copper bracelet at one time, while another survey found they were rarely used. While there is no proof that they work, these bracelets are not harmful.

---

them undesirable for many. Some experts now believe that sleep and arthritis pain are related. In fact, frequent wakings or insomnia appear to be a consequence of arthritis pain or arthritis medications.

Take fibromyalgia, the second most common arthritis-related ailment, for example. As I explain in *The Fibromyalgia Handbook*, stages 3 and 4 of sleep are most important with fibromyalgia (FMS). In these deep stages of sleep, there are large, slow brain waves (delta waves), absent eye movements, and reduced muscle tension. However, we don't know if the sleep problems cause the fibromyalgia symptoms, or if they are secondary to the disease itself. In one study, researchers found that when healthy subjects were deprived of deep sleep because of noise, they experienced musculo-skeletal discomfort and mood symptoms similar to those of the patients with fibromyalgia. These studies suggest that stage 4 sleep disturbance caused the appearance of achiness or pain and mood symptoms.

I've found that most people with arthritis pain need more rest than those without arthritis. A healthy adult may get by with six hours sleep at night, but someone with arthritis needs eight or nine hours to make it through the next day. Melatonin is one dietary supplement that helps patients with sleep problems, it is not readily availiable over the counter in the UK, but it is possible to order it over the internet. This natural hormone, often called the "hormone of darkness," since its secretion is activated almost immediately after exposure to darkness, is produced in the pea-size pineal gland in the center of the brain and regulates the body's circadian rhythms (daily rhythms such as your sleep-wake cycle). In most people, melatonin can give improved sleep, although it can cause grogginess the next day if you are sensitive to it. Most of my patients prefer the time-released melatonin and find it gives them an even dose throughout the night as opposed to a burst of the hormone right at bedtime. Some studies say melatonin raises levels of serotonin, which causes a calming feeling and aids in sound sleep.

If you try melatonin, take a low dose (1 milligram) to start. It may take a few days to get used to this sleep aid, but in most cases, this natural supplement does give benefit.

SAM-e

Although it is not widely availiable in the UK, preliminary study results behind SAM-e (S-adenosyl methionine) are quite promising, as it is thought to have anti-inflammatory, pain-relieving, and tissue-healing properties. At least one large study of SAM-e found similar benefit to naproxen, a common nonsteroid anti-inflammatory drug prescribed to relieve arthritis pain and inflammation. Yet, unlike naproxen or other NSAIDs, SAM-e has few side effects. During clinical trials of SAM-e as a treatment for depression, some patients reported marked improvement in their osteoarthritis.

In studies, researchers believe that SAM-e raises levels of the neuro-transmitter dopamine, which is vital for mood regulation. According to research, SAM-e is not as powerful as St. John's wort, though the mood elevation and anti-inflammatory effects are felt in the body within days. European doctors have prescribed SAM-e for more than twenty years for depression and arthritis pain. I sometimes recommend SAM-e to patients who cannot tolerate NSAIDs and who have mild arthritis pain. Many are able to maintain an active lifestyle using this natural supplement and can avoid the added expense (and side effects) of stronger medications. SAM-e also helps ease anxiety and boost healing, stage 4 sleep—two added benefits to those people who have a chronic illness. (Dosage is 400 milligrams to 1,200 milligrams a day for arthritis.)

Bromelain

A natural protein-digesting enzyme found in pineapple has an anti-inflammatory effect in the body. In uncontrolled studies, bromelain supplements were found to give some relief to rheumatoid arthritis patients, including reduced pain and swelling.

Bromelain works in the body by inhibiting the release of certain inflammation-causing chemicals. It is available in tablet or capsule form for supplemental use. Papaya contains an enzyme called papain that helps the body break down protein, and it is useful to decrease inflammation. Both bromelain and papaya supplements can be found at most drug or health food stores and should be taken bucally (dissolved between your gum and the inside of your cheek).

Essential Fatty Acids

Essential fatty acids (EFAs) are necessary to the immune system because they reduce inflammation by lowering the body's production of prostaglandins. EFAs are available in oils containing omega-3 (fish oils) and omega-6 (linolenic and gamma-linolenic, GLA), which are found in plant oils such as evening primrose, blackcurrant, and borage.

In the past, the omega-3 fatty acids, eicosapentaenoic acid (EPA) and docosahexaenoic acid (DHA) in fish oil have been used primarily for rheumatoid arthritis, which involves significant inflammation, and EPA and DHA have anti-inflammatory effects. However, osteoarthritis also has a degree of inflammation, so EPA may help to reduce this.

It is important to use EPA in addition to your basic treatment program, not to replace it. When used in doses on the label, no serious side effects are known. These fatty acids enable the body to make more products that tend to decrease the inflammation. Eicosapentaenoic acid is available in capsules without a prescription at your drug store or health food store. It takes twelve to sixteen weeks of omega-3 therapy before benefits begin.

Vegetarians who want to gain this anti-inflammatory benefit can substitute flaxseeds or flaxseed oil.

Celadrin

Another dietary supplement called celadrin is thought to help some with knee flexibility and function. Celadrin, composed of concentrated fatty acids, was shown in a small study to alleviate pain and stiffness and increase joint flexibility. In fact, researchers said those who took the supplement for two months were able to walk longer than those taking a placebo.

Gelatin

Findings presented at the 2000 meeting of the Academy of Family Physicians suggested that adding a gelatin supplement to the diet could provide some relief to people with mild osteoarthritis of the knee. In the research, 175 people with osteoarthritis of the knee were given either gelatin supplements or placebo. Those volunteers who took 10 grams of

Good as Gold?

In a two-year study of 55 rheumatoid arthritis patients published in the *Annals of the Rheumatic Diseases*, researchers found that the 30 patients wearing gold wedding bands were less arthritic in the finger joints of that hand than the 25 patients who did not wear gold bands. I don't want you to change your wedding band, but it shows how treatment for arthritis does not always have to come in a prescription bottle!

the gelatin supplement along with vitamin C and calcium reported great reduction in pain and stiffness, and improvement in mobility. While experts are quick to question this study, some believe vitamin C was instrumental in reducing osteoarthritis pain. Vitamin C, a powerful antioxidant and healing nutrient, has been shown in studies to slow the progression of osteoarthritis in some patients.

Super Malic

Malic acid, derived from the food you eat, may play a key role in energy production, especially for those with arthritis and related diseases. In several studies, patients with FMS and other types of arthritis took malic acid. Within forty-eight hours of supplementation, almost all had reduction in pain. Likewise, upon discontinuation of malic acid, the improvement was quickly lost.

Super Malic, a tablet containing malic acid (200 mg) and magnesium (50 mg), is being studied for treatment of fibromyalgia or deep muscle pain and overall aching. In scientific studies, volunteers with FMS took a fixed dose of Super Malic. No symptom change was seen in short-term trials, but when the dose was increased (up to six tablets of Super Malic, twice a day) and continued for a longer duration of treatment in the open-label trial, some reductions in the severity of pain and tenderness were found. (An open-label trial is one in which the medication is not blinded, meaning the drug is known to both the investigator and the participant.)

Sulfur Baths and Mud Packs

Hot sulfur baths and mud packs, given for two weeks at a spa, produced less pain and stiffness, and improvement in patient ease in performing daily tasks, according to a recent study. No severe side effects were found.

In another study from Ben Gurion University, reported in the August 2002 issue of the *Journal of Clinical Rheumatology*, researchers concluded that arthritis patients treated with mud compresses taken from the mineral-rich Dead Sea had less knee pain from osteoarthritis and that this therapy might supplement medical treatment for relief of knee arthritis pain. In the study, very few patients treated with mud without minerals reported improvement.

Researchers believe that Super Malic is safe and may be helpful in treating arthritis and fibromyalgia. If you try Super Malic with your doctor's consent, consider staying on this therapy for at least two months to receive full benefit. (Apples provide both malic acid and magnesium, so include these natural fruits in your daily diet for a possible pain benefit.)

Homeopathy

Another natural complement to conventional medicine is homeopathy, a two-hundred-year-old medical system commonly used in Europe, Asia, and Latin America. In fact, homeopathy is the most frequently used alternative therapy in the world.

By selecting the correct homeopathic medicine from the plant, mineral, animal, or chemical source, practitioners believe you can stimulate your body's own defenses rather than suppress symptoms. Homeopathy is based on the Law of Similars, which states that any substance that can cause symptoms when given to healthy people can also heal those who are experiencing similar symptoms. For instance, radiation can cause cancer, yet it is also used as a cancer treatment. Gold can successfully treat arthritis, yet it can also cause joint pain.

With homeopathy, medications are diluted so that toxic properties are minimized and potential healing properties are magnified. This pharmaceutical process is called *potentization,* or successive dilution. It is the combined process of dilution and vigorous shaking that makes the medicine effective. Some commonly used homeopathic remedies include *Bryonia alba, Pulsatilla nigricans,* and *Rhus toxicodendron.*

Although some small studies have been performed using homeopathic treatments, there is no firm conclusion as to the effectiveness of homeopathic remedies in the treatment of arthritis.

Use Caution with Some Supplements

Not all supplements ease pain—even if the package labeling makes that claim. I would avoid or use caution with the following supplements until further research confirms that they are safe to use and have proven results.

Arthritis 101

At this point, some discussion of the "placebo response phenomenon" is necessary. Placebo is Latin for "I shall please" (the opening phrase of the Catholic vespers for the dead, an ironic reference in the original coining of the word). Placebos are usually viewed as inactive treatments (sugar pills) that doctors give merely to "please" anxious patients or to indulge insatiable ones. However, it has been shown that the placebo effect yields beneficial effects in 60 to 90 percent of diseases that include angina pectoris, bronchial asthma, herpes simplex, and duodenal ulcer. Three elements are involved in this effect:

1. Positive belief and expectations by the patient
2. Positive belief and expectations by the physician or health care provider
3. A good relationship between the two parties

Interestingly, some interventions that can be considered placebo, unreal, or inert turn out to produce various biochemical or physiologic changes. While not everyone responds to placebos, it is reported that 30 to 40 percent of those treated responded to placebo, with up to 55 percent responding in terms of pain relief. Unfortunately, there is no way to select a consistent "placebo responder."

D-Phenylalanine

D-phenylalanine is a synthetic variation of the amino acid L-phenylalanine and is said to reduce osteoarthritis pain. Some believe that a few amino acids, including D-phenylalanine (DPA), actually increase tolerance to pain by blocking the enzymes that break down endorphins and enkephalins, the body's natural pain-killing chemicals. Until there is more substantive research on this amino acid, it may be a waste of your money to try it.

New Zealand Green-Lipped Mussel

New Zealand green-lipped mussel (*Perna canaliculus*) has been used for decades as an alternative therapy for those with arthritis pain, but I've yet to see solid evidence that it helps alleviate pain without the risk of side effects such as upset stomach, gout, and skin rashes. For now, I'd hold off on this alternative therapy, even if your neighbor recommends it. From my experience, those who most recommend green-lipped mussel are those who are selling it!

DMSO

DMSO has been used for years in the treatment of muscle strains and sprains in horses. It's also used in humans for treatment of some bladder diseases. It has been used with some benefit in the treatment of injuries to muscles and tendons, especially athletic injuries. In injuries, DMSO is applied to the painful area (not taken internally).

In the past decade, DMSO has become a popular treatment for arthritis. An impure form of DMSO is sold in hardware and other stores, which many have used instead of the pure form. When applied to the skin, DMSO penetrates and is absorbed into the blood. It causes a breath odor somewhat like garlic that is distinctive. The skin may become irritated where it is used.

The use of DMSO for therapeutic applications is controversial. While some research shows that DMSO has anti-inflammatory properties and alleviates pain when rubbed into the skin, there is also the risk of toxicity when the impure form is used or if it is used too frequently. If your doctor approves DMSO and it's used under a doctor's supervision, it may be helpful to some with arthritis pain. But at this time, I do not recommend the use of DMSO until further studies are made and it is approved as both safe and effective.

Vinegar and Honey

One alternative therapy that has been around for decades is the folk medicine belief that people with arthritis don't produce enough acid in their stomachs. Apple cider vinegar is used to provide the acid. When the vinegar is ingested (in a glass of water), it is said to make the tissues less tender, more elastic, improve the disposition, help constipation, improve the health of the skin, prevent growth of harmful germs, change the blood flow to the digestive organs, and other actions. Vinegar and water are also used to soak the hands and feet.

Honey is used in the treatment of arthritis and other problems in some older alternative cures. Honey is said to improve digestion, relieve pain in arthritis, attract fluid, help the body to destroy harmful germs, provide nutrients, have a laxative effect, and have the effect of a sedative. The honey is mixed in water with apple cider vinegar and ingested at meals or other times.

Iodine and kelp tablets are also part of the treatment of arthritis, according to some natural health followers. When used in moderate amounts, there is no evidence that any of these nutritional treatments are harmful. Some people feel more peace of mind after they have tried this sort of treatment, just in case it helps the arthritis pain.

NADH

NADH (nicotinamide adenine dinucleotide) is a naturally occurring coenzyme nutrient found in all living cells. This enzyme plays a central role in the body's energy-producing capacity. There is ongoing research using NADH to treat patients with chronic fatigue. Researchers at Georgetown University treated patients with chronic fatigue syndrome with NADH with promising results. Patients reported relief from fatigue, along with increased strength and endurance, and a boost in mental and physical energy.

Although the studies are not conclusive, NADH may help those who suffer with inattentiveness or daytime fatigue because of arthritis or fibromyalgia pain. Stay on top of the news for more information before you decide to take this natural dietary supplement. For now, NADH is unproven and extremely expensive.

Magnet Therapy

Many people with arthritis turn to magnet therapy as an alternative treatment to pharmaceuticals. Magnet therapy is not new; Hippocrates and Paracelsus practiced magnet therapy in the Middle Ages. Today, well-known athletes use this drugless therapy for relieving pain and claim on infomercials to get relief within minutes. It is believed that the magnet somehow stimulates or interacts with the body's electrical system to increase circulation, reduce inflammation, and decrease pain. Some believe the magnets stimulate endorphins (natural painkillers) in the body.

It will take subsequent studies to make any guarantees about magnet therapy for arthritis pain. At this time, the National Institute of Health has created an office of alternative medicine that is paying for the magnet studies on fibromyalgia patients at the University of Virginia.

The downside of magnet therapy is the unknown. According to the U.S. Food and Drug Administration, magnets marketed with medical claims are considered medical devices because they are promoted to treat a medical condition. The FDA warns doctors about the unknown side effects of magnet therapy. Just as they do not know if magnets can end

Let's Review: 8 Steps to Getting Started with Alternative Therapies

1. Talk to your doctor for approval to try alternative therapies. Stay on your prescribed medications. Make sure there will be no drug-herb interaction.
2. Be selective when choosing a natural dietary supplement and stick with the known brands.
3. Make sure you understand how to read the label on natural dietary supplements, as explained on page 70. If in doubt, talk to your pharmacist or physician.
4. If you take herbs such as feverfew or white willow bark, be sure to stop any other anti-inflammatory medication such as aspirin or ibuprofen. (Make sure your doctor approves.)
5. If you take an herb to help induce sleep, be sure there are no interactions with other sleep aids. Talk to your doctor.
6. If you are allergic to shellfish, avoid glucosamine.
7. If you find relief from an age-old remedy such as a copper bracelet, wear one. I believe that it is hard to discourage use if someone feels a safe therapy really works.
8. Continue with all steps of the Pain-Free Program for optimal relief.

pain, they don't know if they are harmful, either. Some patients have reported such side effects as headaches, insomnia, and backache after extensive magnet therapy.

It's important to realize that though there is hope for magnet therapy in stopping chronic pain, it is still highly experimental and has been reported, if used incorrectly, to induce seizures in healthy people. Don't use magnet therapy if you have a cardiac pacemaker.

Doctor's Alternative Treatment

Whatever therapy you choose, it's important to take responsibility for your own health—understand your illness and learn all you can about the various methods, including alternative or natural therapies, to treat it. Be sure to talk to your doctor before taking any unproven herbal treatment or dietary supplement, and do not stop your prescribed medication unless advised by your doctor. Also, let your doctor know about all medications you take to ensure that the supplement will not counteract the effectiveness of the drug or have a toxic effect in the body.

Osteoarthritis
- Valerian (page 75) may help you get to sleep easier, especially on days when you have more pain.
- Glucosamine (page 76) helps many with mild to moderate osteoarthritis pain. Follow package instructions.
- Essential fatty acids (EFAs) can reduce inflammation (page 79).

Fibromyalgia
- Melatonin (page 77) or valerian (page 75) may help if you have trouble sleeping.
- SAM-e (page 78) might ease anxiety and depression, boost sound sleep, and may also help ease the deep muscle pain.
- Magnesium supplementation (page 48) may help to lessen deep muscle pain. Ask your doctor to see if it might be helpful in your situation.
- Super Malic (page 81) works in relieving pain in some with FMS.

Rheumatoid Arthritis (and Other Inflammatory Arthritis)
- EPA—fish oil—capsules (page 79) can ease inflammation. If you are a vegetarian, try flaxseed oil.
- Arnica or capsaicin rubs (page 75) used on painful joints can help to ease pain.
- Glucosamine may give relief for inflammatory arthritis. Try this supplement, but if you find no relief after two to three weeks, discontinue use.

Gout
- The over-the-counter supplement quercetin is a highly concentrated form of bioflavonoid and has been found to reduce the pain and inflammation of gout. Follow package label for dosage.

Make Key Lifestyle Changes

When I speak to groups, I often get the question, "What can I do to protect my joints from further injury?" In many situations, making a few lifestyle adjustments can help to protect your joints, prevent further injury, and even stop pain altogether. For instance, I have one patient, Rachel, a fifty-three-year-old computer programmer with osteoarthritis, whose hip pain kept her from sleeping well and prevented exercise. After trying several medications without much luck, I suggested that she get a different chair to see if the way she was sitting might place undue stress on her painful arthritic hip. Within one week of trying the new chair, she

Gather Your Pain-Free Tools

1. In your Pain-Free Diary, write down specific changes that work for you as you read this step—including ways to protect your joints, arrange your daily tasks, and revamp areas in your home that may increase your risk for falling.
2. Using the suggestions in this chapter, record necessary changes you must make throughout your home and workplace to increase safety and reduce the chance of falling.
3. Make a list of special tools that may help you when arthritis pain flares. Check the Resources section at the end of the book for websites that market these arthritis aids.
4. Write down specific tips on gardening, travel, sleep, and intimacy and incorporate these in your daily life, so you can do the things you enjoy.

called and said her hip pain had greatly diminished. Another patient, Ron, owns a small retail store. Ron had to relearn how to properly lift heavy boxes but in doing so, he also ended lower back pain that had plagued him for more than three years.

Organize for Pain-Free Living

You are more than halfway through with the Pain-Free Program, and I hope you're feeling confident as you start each step. Now that you've

---

Wear Shoes That Fit

Be sure your shoes are not adding to your pain. Inappropriate shoes increase the risk of callus and ulcer formation, as well as increase the risk of falls. For arthritis pain in the feet or ankles, shoes can give extra support and make walking easier. Nevertheless, if shoes are too tight or if there are areas of excess pressure then the feet can be an extra source of pain. Studies by the American Academy of Orthopedic Surgeons show that 43 million Americans have foot problems, which costs the nation more than $3.5 billion a year. A revealing survey of 1,724 people by this same organization found that 80 percent of women said their feet hurt; almost 60 percent said they wore uncomfortable shoes at least an hour each day.

So, what kind of shoe is best? In a comprehensive study published in the April 2001 issue of the *Lancet*, researchers reported that chunky heels on high-heeled shoes are just as bad on your knees as the stiletto heels, increasing pressure on the inside of the knee. I recommend that patients change to a sturdy flat shoe in order to decrease knee pain and be active again. Studies show that most women wear their shoes too small—which can greatly increase pressure on the feet and ankles, resulting in damage. That's why to end pain you need to wear shoes that support your weight yet don't put abnormal pressure on joints. When your weight distribution is improved, excess forces on the knees and hips are reduced and pain diminishes.

If you have arthritis in your feet, it would be worthwhile to see a podiatrist (foot doctor). Depending on your type of pain, your doctor may prescribe orthotics or a specially designed insert to put inside your shoe, helping to alleviate heel or ankle pain. Specialty shoe stores have these available and the insert is made specifically for your foot and problem.

reviewed Steps 1 to 3, I want you to consider making some key lifestyle changes that will help reduce your pain and stiffness. In Step 4, you will learn how to arrange your daily tasks, including dressing, eating, picking up heavy items, and bending or stooping. I'll also guide you in reworking your living quarters to help you avoid falling—one of the biggest causes of injuries at home and one that will greatly aggravate your pain. First, let me tell you about Madeline.

Madeline is a forty-three-year-old physical education teacher and former professional dancer. When she was diagnosed with osteoarthritis of the ankles last year, I was surprised that her X rays showed so much joint deterioration. Madeline did ballet on point for years, traveling abroad with different ballet companies. Now, at midlife, all the years of constant weight bearing on her ankles has resulted in wear and tear on her joints. This fairly young woman was concerned that because her ankles were weak and painful, she'd lose her balance and trip, resulting in even more pain or a possible fracture.

I explained to Madeline that athletes and dancers were at higher risk of getting osteoarthritis early in life, even as young as thirty or forty. Now she needed to start the Pain-Free Program with exercises to strengthen the muscles around her ankles, and make some easy lifestyle changes to diminish the risk of tripping or falling. I also encouraged Madeline to learn tai chi, which is an effective way to prevent falls in adults. Because of the slow, graceful body movements, tai chi helps to improve balance and flexibility. Tai chi works for all ages. In one study, those who practiced tai chi reduced their risk of falls by about 40 percent.

So far in this book you've learned why exercise is vital to keep muscles strong, joints flexible, and reduce pain. You have also learned to work with your particular type of arthritis and lose weight, if necessary, as well as add key nutrients to reduce inflammation and increase healing. I've given you important information on natural dietary supplements that can ease pain and, in some cases, allowed you to cut back on medications. Now, in this fourth step, I want to give you crucial advice for making simple lifestyle changes that can let you live pain-free.

Here are the four overall goals of Step 4:

1. To implement the Fall-Proof Plan, which you can start today
2. To show ways to protect arthritic joints from further pain or injury
3. To help you become the master of your pain before it takes control of you

4. To give helpful tips on gardening, travel, sleep, and sex so you can continue to enjoy your life

With Step 4, you will achieve these goals and begin to realize the optimal benefit of living pain-free. Let's first address how to implement my Fall-Proof Plan at home.

Pain-Free Strategy #1: Implement the Fall-Proof Plan

You've heard the adage, "If you fail to plan, you plan to fail." For the sake of the Pain-Free Program, let's modify those words to be: *"If you fail to plan, you plan to FALL."* It only takes one careless fall to set you up for months of pain and immobility.

Falling is the most common home injury and is second to motor vehicle crashes as the most common cause of death from all accidental injuries. According to the Home Safety Network in the UK, nearly 4,000 people in Britain die each year from falling down stairwells, tripping over lamp cords, and other accidents inside their homes. There are many reasons people fall—from dim lighting to poor balance to bad eyesight to medications that may cause dizziness or weakness. I've had patients fall because of poorly fitting shoes, loose objects such as furniture or rugs, and lack of bathroom safety equipment during painful arthritis flares.

However, for those with arthritis, any fall can be devastating, adding further injury to the inflamed joints and sore muscles, intensifying your pain and sometimes causing fractures that put you out of commission for

---

Protect Your Joints

- Depend on your larger joints to do the work of smaller joints. For instance, ask for plastic bags when grocery shopping. Instead of carrying the heavy bag with your fingers and hand, hang the bag over your arm. This simple maneuver moves the weight of the bag to the shoulder and upper body and eliminates unnecessary stress on delicate joints in the hand or wrist.
- Plan ahead. If you are doing laundry, gather all items and put into one basket. Then, carry these down the stairs or hallway to the laundry room. If you are preparing dinner, put all ingredients on the countertop before you begin cooking.

months. That is why my Fall-Proof Plan can help you avoid further pain problems. Use the following safety tips as you continue the Pain-Free Program. (You will not need to follow every suggestion; just select the ones that fit in your own situation.)

Fall-Proof the Home Entry

Many people fall when they step out of their cars and begin the short walk to their homes. One of my patients with osteoarthritis of the hip tripped over the garden hose one night and ended up with a hip fracture—in the same arthritic hip. Another patient with osteoarthritis of the spine tripped over a sidewalk stepping-stone and was hospitalized for a fractured vertebra. Can you imagine the unnecessary pain both patients suffered, not to mention the months of inconvenient rehabilitation? Yet, there is a way to avoid these mishaps altogether.

First, keep garden hoses coiled when not in use and tuck them next to the house. Some garden hoses automatically recoil when not in use, which can save you time and decrease your risk of tripping. Also, make sure the sidewalk is level leading to the front door. I cannot tell you how many patients have tripped on a sidewalk crack or uneven cement.

The entrance doormat should lie flat on the ground and have no turned-up or frayed edges. If children or grandchildren have balls, bikes, or other toys in the yard, make sure these are stored properly immediately after use. Most important is proper lighting during evening hours so the walkway is clearly visible.

Fall-Proof the Living Room

After tripping on a piece of loose carpet, forty-one-year-old Camille finally took seriously the need to fall-proof her home. This mother of three has had rheumatoid arthritis for years, and on days when her RA flares even hugging her children is painful. The fall on the loose carpet set Camille back a few months in the Pain-Free Program. Just when she was beginning to feel energized and her RA symptoms were well managed, the fall caused her to hurt again for days, and she had to cancel a business trip to London with her husband.

Make sure your living room gets a thorough fall-proof evaluation. The entrance should be free of obstructions, such as slippery tiles or frayed rugs. Check the living room lighting and make sure it is adequate. Studies show that as we age, we need two to three times as much illumination as young adults. Also, make sure there are no telephone cords or lamp cords

---

Protect Your Knees

- Keep your knees flexible so you can straighten the knees completely when you walk. It is much more work and pressure on the knee cartilage to stand or walk when the knee is slightly bent. Try walking with your knees slightly bent, and notice the difference.
- If you have to stand for long periods, put your leg on a stool or chair, and rest the knees for a few minutes two or three times a day with your knee straight.
- Avoid propping your knees on pillows when you sleep. This causes the knees to stay in a bent position, making it more difficult to straighten. But, if you sleep on your side (fetal position), you may find more pain relief with a pillow between the knees. Stretch your knees in the morning before walking.
- Use joint warmers, which fit around the knee, for warmth and to help with stability.
- Avoid stairs and steps at home.

---

in walkways, and hem any drapes or curtains that are too long and could cause a potential problem.

Make certain that tables, chairs, and couches are the proper height (your hips should never be lower than your knees). Anchor the rugs so they cannot be lifted (get carpet strips at any home or carpet store), and feel the carpet for raised spots that might throw you off balance.

Fall-Proof the Stairway and Hallway

"One fall down the stairs did this to me." Kent showed me his bruised, swollen ankles, as he told of hurrying down the stairs in his socks, trying to make his car pool for work. Now this fifty-year-old stockbroker was homebound until the ankle joints healed.

Make sure your stairs are well lighted and have a solid banister or railing on both sides. Hold on to this railing when going up and down and take one step at a time, if you need to. (It's easiest to go up steps, leading with your better side.) Always wear shoes when using the stairs. When Kent's socks slid on the wooden stairs, he lost control because he had no traction. Slow down, and take each step cautiously to avoid falling.

Remove any clutter or throw rugs that could block the walkway of the stairs. Put bright, contrasting colored tape on the top and bottom steps. This will serve as a reminder to use with caution. If you're using the stairs at bedtime, make sure your robe or pajamas are not too long so as to cause you to trip. Put a small basket or plastic carrier off to the side of the stairs to put items in to carry up and down, so you can still hold on to the banister.

Fall-Proof the Bathroom

The bathroom is the most dangerous place in the home for falls, yet there are many easy changes you can make to ensure safety. First, purchase a raised toilet seat that fits on top of the regular toilet. Also, install lever handles on the sink, if you have arthritis in the hands. These handles are easier to maneuver and put less force on your hand joints.

Purchase a rubber bath mat that runs the length of the tub and has a nonslip surface. You might find a nonskid stool with a back useful. You can put this in the tub for moist heat treatments. You might consider a water-resistant and height-adjustable "bath bench" or chair. This bench lets you sit at a normal height in the bathtub while bathing and is safe for moist heat applications. Using the self-help products websites in the Resources section, look for a specially designed bath sponge that is attached to a long pliable handle. This will allow you to bend it and wash your back with minimal effort. A handheld showerhead can be vertically mounted with a sliding bar to give you easy access to the shower. Tools such as this can keep you from losing your balance during bathing.

Install grab bars on walls around the tub and beside the toilet. Soap dishes or towel rods can break away under a person's weight. Make sure the grab bars are strong enough to support your weight. Also, make sure the floor has a nonskid surface with carpeting or a nonskid bath mat.

Fall-Proof the Kitchen

The kitchen is another common area for falls, especially as people try to get items that are out of their reach or lose their balance and slip on wet floors. You can avoid mishaps in your kitchen if you take a few fall-proof steps.

First, never use a stepstool or ladder to put an item in a high cabinet or to retrieve an item. Keep all dishes, cookware, and food items within reach. If you must get an item from a higher shelf, purchase pickup tongs (about 2 feet in length) to grab the item, and lower it to the countertop (see websites in the Resources section). Better still, ask someone to get the item for you.

Put cabinet or pantry shelves on casters so the items are easy to access. You can also have someone install pull-out shelves. A pegboard is an attractive way to store pots and other utensils. On the other hand, some people like to hang pots and pans from easy-to-access decorative hooks. (Your local kitchen supply store has an array of options from which to choose.)

Make sure the pots and utensils have easy grab handles, so you do not strain your wrist during the cooking process—important for those with arthritis in their hands or wrists. You can reduce the forces on your hand joints by supporting the wrist that's lifting the object with your other wrist. To avoid carrying a heavy pot across the kitchen and risking a fall, use a cart with wheels to move items around the kitchen.

Again, as with all rooms in your home, make sure the kitchen lighting is bright, using the highest wattage bulb your system can handle.

Fall-Proof the Bedroom

Unbelievably, simply getting out of bed has landed a few of my patients in the emergency room. Jack, a middle-aged man with ankylosing spondylitis, slipped on the bedspread getting out of bed in the middle of the night and fractured a vertebra in his spine. Another woman, Lynne, tripped on her bed's dust ruffle and fell on her arthritic knee. These mishaps do *not* have to happen to you.

First, make sure your bedroom lighting is adequate, especially at nighttime. Have a reliable light next to your bed, and leave a closet light on at night or have a nightlight in the hallway. Put a flashlight in your nightstand in case of power outage or if you still have trouble seeing at night.

Now walk around your bed and remove all clutter. Make sure your bedspread or comforter fits tightly and does not slip off the bed. The dust ruffle should be off the floor. If you have wood floors, do not use a cleaner that adds shine to avoid creating a slippery surface. Never use decorative rugs next to your bed, as these can easily slip. If needed, get a bed rail that helps you balance as you get in and out of bed (see the Resources section).

Remember, these proactive fall-proofing steps will allow you to avoid mishaps that could undo all your progress with the Pain-Free Program. It will just take an hour or two to ensure your optimal safety—and the long-term results will be well worth it.

Pain-Free Strategy #2: Become the Master of Your Pain

To stop arthritis from taking over your life, it's important to take control and become the master of your pain. If you are overly committed with volunteer commitments or career, the chances are great that you'll have a more difficult time managing your arthritis and pain. In this pain-free strategy, I want to show how you can put yourself at the top of your daily To Do list using the following steps, or POD:

1. Pace yourself.
2. Organize.
3. Delegate.

One of my patients, Beth, a retired English teacher, recommended the acronym POD, saying it helped her to remember the three key steps of this strategy. This sixty-seven-year-old woman has the combination of rheumatoid arthritis and fibromyalgia—both extremely painful ailments. Yet Beth lives an amazingly active life, serving as president of her condo association, volunteering three days a week at a nearby elementary school, and teaching art classes at a local community center. Even though Beth is busy and productive, her arthritis is well controlled. She has become the master of her pain as she carefully schedules her time, prioritizes her commitments, and asks for help from family and friends. In order to live an active life with a chronic, painful ailment, here is what Beth and others have learned using POD.

Pace Yourself

Just because your spouse can stay up all hours of the night and still feel energetic the next day does not always mean you can. Having a chronic, painful illness puts an extra burden on you physically, mentally, and emotionally. In addition, you must allow for this by always conserving your energy. Here are some suggestions:

- If you plan to go to dinner, schedule a period of rest beforehand.
- If you have a busy outing planned, make sure you have no plans the night before so you can allow your body to rest.
- If you have an upcoming business meeting or presentation, block your calendar to allow for plenty of rest the night before.
- After all-day outings or late-night gatherings, block your calendar for a few days so you can recover from the busyness and activity.

• If you're feeling especially tired and achy, cancel the outing or activity altogether. Rather than push yourself and live with the consequences of exhaustion and more pain, wait until you feel rested, are pain-free, and have more energy.

Be creative and think of ways to accomplish tasks that require less effort. For instance, the assistive devices listed in this step may let you accomplish tasks without a lot of energy and with much less pain. After work, do your household or yard chores in short "bursts" instead of all at once. For instance, you might do the following:

• Vacuum and change bed linens on Monday.
• Clean bathrooms on Tuesday.
• Mop on Wednesday.
• Dust on Thursday.
• Clean out the refrigerator and pantry on Friday.
• Do yard work on Saturday.
• Rest on Sunday.

Breaking large jobs into small, doable tasks lets you get the work done but also allows time for rest in between, so you can feel well enough to enjoy your home and family. *Never* work to the point of fatigue. If you are like most arthritis patients, doing so will take its toll and you'll pay for it later on with sheer exhaustion and increased pain and stiffness. Before you tackle a household or yard project, take time to apply moist heat and warm up with some stretching. If the project is taxing, take a

Protect Your Hips

• Keep the hips flexible so you can fully straighten them.
• Use a cane in the hand on the opposite side of your arthritic hip. Be sure the length is correct for your height and the handle fits your hand.
• Sleep or lie on your stomach for 30 minutes or more each day to help prevent deformity in the hips.
• Avoid stairs and steps at home.
• If you fall frequently and have osteoporosis, consider hip protectors. They can lower the risk of hip fracture by 50 percent.

warm bath or shower when you are finished to help decrease pain and stiffness.

Organize

In your Pain-Free Diary, make a list of all the commitments you have each week. Include current obligations—work, family commitments, and community involvement. Be sure to include on this list your twice-daily moist heat applications, exercise, and periods for rest. Now, when you start adding to your list a host of volunteer commitments, evening meetings, career obligations, or other activities, you could face overload resulting in additional stress. You need to select where to draw the line— and no one can draw this line but you.

After you have completed your list of activities and commitments, prioritize these, and divide this list into two sections: Section 1 will be those commitments that you cannot change or *Essential Tasks*; section 2 will be those that are more flexible or *Additional Tasks*, which you can choose to do or not.

After you prioritize your list of commitments, cross out those that are not crucial to your health or well-being. What changes can you make in your list of priorities? Work on what you can change (list 2, *Additional Tasks*), and accept what you can't change (list 1, *Essential Tasks*). Just be sure to stay on top of the time spent on all commitments so that your main priority tasks get done each day.

Now number the items on list 1 (*Essential Tasks*) in order of their priority so you can become more focused and attend to the items that must receive your attention first. Some people find that crossing off each item as they complete it gives them a sense of accomplishment. Divide large tasks that seem overwhelming into smaller parts that can be accomplished in more realistic time slots, and complete one at a time. Start with item 1 on your *Essential Tasks* list at the most productive time of the day. Choose the time when you feel the least pain and your mind is most clear. That will enable you to focus and really get your responsibilities accomplished.

As you prioritize your list of commitments, set reasonable expectations. A constant push for perfection can cause undue stress, which results in hazards to our mental and physical well-being. Researchers are learning that perfectionism may be a key risk factor in burnout. Some of these commitments are bound to be making dents in your schedule and are significant wasters of your valuable time.

No Rain, No Pain!

Although difficult to prove because we don't have a "pain barometer," most of my arthritis patients are greatly affected by changes in the weather. Some new findings in February 2002 in the *Journal of Rheumatology* support this, concluding that cooler temperatures, high humidity, and high or low atmospheric pressure may be associated with spontaneous pain among individuals with arthritis or fibromyalgia. I have seen decreases in barometric pressure increase pain in my patients with osteoarthritis. You may have noticed that decreases in barometric pressure cause an increase in pain, making it harder to exercise or be active. Some patients report more pain when there are rapid changes up or down in barometric pressure.

Scientists know that when barometric pressure decreases, the wall tension of an arterial vessel decreases, allowing the vessel to expand. Some researchers believe that this vascular expansion contributes to the increased pain arthritis patients feel during weather changes.

If you know a weather front is approaching, make sure you are taking your arthritis medication and continue the twice-daily moist heat soaks or applications. Stretching and range-of-motion exercises should also help you to avoid stiffness or increased pain.

Delegate

You have every right to ask for help when needed and delegate tasks that may stress your body. On days when your arthritis flares, ask family members, friends, or co-workers to fill in or help you accomplish a task. On days when you are pain-free, return the favor, and let them know you appreciate their willingness to help. Get family members to do chores that might increase your pain, such as carrying the garbage to the curb, mowing the lawn, or vacuuming. Affirm their willingness to pitch in, and return the favor in another way, as you are able. If you cannot count on friends or family members, consider hiring outside help for cleaning or yard work.

Pain-Free Strategy 3: Start to Enjoy Your Life Again

"Just knowing that I have control over my arthritis releases the fears and anxiety for me. When I first got the diagnosis, I thought I'd have to give up doing the things I enjoyed. Now I realize that my life can be active and full, if I learn how to stay pain-free." Most patients are relieved when

I explain that arthritis does not mean they have to sit on the sidelines in life. With daily exercise, moist heat, proper weight and diet, and other strategies in the Pain-Free Program, almost all men and women can continue their active lives—with a few simple modifications. Fifty-year-old Beth, a librarian with rheumatoid arthritis and chronic lung disease, was determined to beat the limitations of chronic illness. With regular exercise, pacing herself, and effective medications to treat both diseases, Beth now plays three sets of tennis at least twice each week and swims a half-mile each day at the local gym.

Here are some suggestions for modifying your activities so you can still enjoy life's simple pleasures.

Gardening Tips

Maybe it's because my practice is on Florida's Gulf coast where the average annual temperature is 72 degrees Fahrenheit, but most of my patients enjoy being outdoors and gardening is a popular hobby. Here are some ways to continue gardening, even with arthritis. You can modify these tips to use in other favorite activities and hobbies.

- *Organize ahead of time.* Make sure you have all your necessary tools and supplies by you when you begin your gardening project. This will conserve your energy so you can complete the task. If you are planting, ask someone to set the heavy bag of soil and container of plants at the site of your garden or put the soil into smaller bags. This will help you to avoid back pain or strain from lifting heavy objects.
- *Avoid kneeling on hard surfaces.* Purchase a thick kneeling pad or stool and put your knees on this instead of the hard ground.
- *Take frequent breaks.* Get up every 10 to 15 minutes and stretch. Walk around before resuming your kneeling position. Staying in one position is likely to make your joints begin to ache and will make it more difficult to straighten the knees and hips.
- *Change your gardening style.* Consider doing container or raised-bed gardening. This keeps you from stooping or bending and still lets you enjoy nature and your favorite plants.
- *Install an irrigation system.* This will keep you from daily watering during dry spells.
- *Check out special equipment.* Some specialty gardening shops have tools with large-grip handles or long handles. These easy-to-grip

hand tools can greatly reduce stress on the wrists and longer handles can keep you from bending.

- *Purchase a gardening cart or wheelbarrow.* Use this to move plants, potting soil, rocks, and other gardening materials. It's easier to move several items by pushing a wheelbarrow than to lift each item and move it individually. Try a lightweight plastic cart that can be mobile and easy to move when necessary.

Travel Tips

You can still travel, even with arthritis. I believe travel to be a superb form of exercise for the body and mind and encourage my patients to take trips. Here are some steps to get you started:

- *Plan ahead.* Choose a destination that fits your type of arthritis. For instance, if you have painful hips or knees, it is probably wise to avoid sightseeing that entails a lot of walking, climbing steps, or hiking. But if you find yourself in one of these situations, use a taxi or a wheelchair if you need to see everything without pain and fatigue.
- *Pack lightly.* Limit your bags to less than twenty-five pounds total weight, and make sure your luggage is on wheels so you can pull it. Limit your carry-on bag to one lightweight shoulder bag. Some travel experts suggest taking half of what you think you might need on the trip, and have clothes laundered in the hotel room to allow for this reduction. Most travelers take more clothes than needed. You don't have to plan for all possible dress occasions each trip!
- *Travel at nonpeak times.* It's easier to access the plane and your luggage if you travel at nonpeak travel times (such as midafternoon). You will also have easier access to rides in an electric cart. Be sure to request the cart when you make your reservation and the airline will ensure its arrival at your gate. When you fly, ask for a bulkhead seat or an aisle seat so you'll have extra room for stretching.
- *Use a wheelchair.* Don't forget that airlines offer wheelchairs for long-distance walking. This can greatly conserve your energy for later enjoyable activities. You will likely find that a wheelchair ride will avoid slowing down your travel or tour group.
- *Get nonstop flights.* Ask your travel agent to make reservations for nonstop flights whenever possible. This lets you avoid changing planes, standing in long lines, walking from gate to gate, and sitting in uncomfortable waiting rooms waiting for a flight.

Protect Your Back

- When you lift an object from the floor, stand close to the object. Start with the center of the weight about 8 inches from your body. Hold the object close to your body instead of at arm's length. (Lifting with the arms held out puts higher amounts of stress on the back.)
- Lift with your legs—not your back. The strength of the legs takes the load off back muscles.
- The distance lifted should be no more than 12 to 13 inches for a weight above 86 pounds. If the weight is heavier, the distance lifted should be shorter. If the object must be lifted higher, then get assistance.
- Avoid lifting objects higher than chest level. Lifting above this level may cause higher stress on the back muscles.
- Lifting the above weight carefully no more than every 5 minutes is recommended. When you must lift more often, be sure you follow the other guidelines to prevent injury.
- Never twist your back when lifting, as it puts more force on the back. If you have to turn, pivot with your feet.
- Always be sure of your footing. A sudden change in foot placement or a trip can cause excess stress on the back.
- If the object to be lifted is too heavy, have someone else help you lift or use a mechanical lever or machine.
- More force is put on the back when you lift using only one hand, so always use two hands when lifting. Sudden lifting, such as jerking the object, also causes a great increase in back pressure. Try to make your lifts smooth and gradual to lower the workload on your back.

- *Bring all medications.* Take all your arthritis medications with you, particularly any prescription medicine, so you won't have to find these items at your destination. Ask your doctor for a small supply of pain medication in case of arthritis flare-ups during travel.
- *Stay active.* If you travel by car, try to stop every one to two hours and walk around—even a short walk around your car can help ease pain and stiffness. Stretch your arms and legs, and gently move your joints in their range of motion. The reduction in your pain and stiffness will be noticeable and will make the small investment in time more than worthwhile. When you travel by airplane or train, walk up and down the aisle several times during the trip. Just a few

minutes of walking or stretching can greatly help the stiffness and tiredness.

- *Choose the right accommodations.* Select a hotel that works best for your type of arthritis. For instance, if stairs make your knees or hips hurt, make sure your hotel has an elevator access or is at ground level. Ask about a heated swimming pool, a Jacuzzi, and an exercise room. You can even continue your exercise program and moist heat, using the shower or bath in your hotel room. If you need ramps or other facilities for wheelchairs, it is a good idea to check with the hotel before you make your reservations. Most now have designated rooms with grab bars in showers, bathtubs, and toilets.
- *Take time to rest.* Allow time during each day to rest. Use this time to lie down or prop your legs on a chair. You can read, watch television, or daydream—but your body is getting that much-needed reprieve so it can continue your active pace. You can rejoin your family or friends later when you are feeling less pain and stiffness.

Intimacy Tips

I have arthritis patients of all ages who stop having sex because of back, shoulder, or hip pain. Martin, a fifty-nine-year-old attorney with osteoarthritis of the hip and knees, confided in me recently that he felt depressed because he no longer could have sex with his wife of thirty-five years. "We used to have a healthy sex life before I got arthritis. I love my wife and want to be intimate, but I'm just afraid the pain will keep me from working the next day."

I encouraged Martin to continue seeking an active sex life instead of falling victim to a chronic illness. Martin is a healthy man with arthritis, and I pointed out the many reasons sex could increase his sense of well-being and diminish his depression. Sex causes the body to release hormones called endorphins, which are the body's own natural painkillers. Many experts believe that endorphins can help to reduce arthritis pain and help you to feel more positive about life. Martin left the clinic that day feeling hopeful that he and his wife could continue with intimacy, finding the right positions and moments that work for their relationship. These are the tips I shared with Martin and other patients on how to continue intimacy in spite of arthritis pain:

- *Find what works for you.* There are many ways to be intimate with the person you love—from holding hands while watching a movie

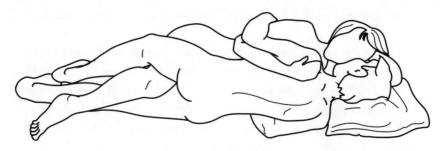

Figure 4.1.

For men with back problems, use the side position with the man and woman facing each other.

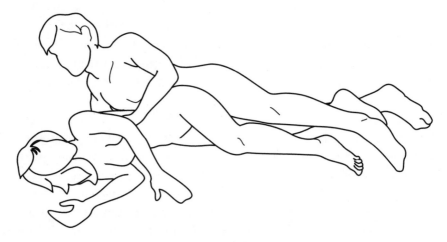

Figure 4.2.

For women with hip problems, use the side position with the man behind. Put a pillow between your knees for stabilizing the body.

to enjoying a gourmet meal together to having sex. During painful flare-ups, you might have to change positions or even resort to just being physically close until the pain resolves. Intimacy is not about performing like those in movies, it's about finding what works for you and makes you both feel close and loved. As some have said, the greatest sex organ is the mind.

• *Explore a variety of positions.* Find the best sexual position with the least discomfort that works best for you and your type of arthritis. Make sure you are comfortable and adjust your body frequently to avoid aches and stiffness. I've given two examples of positions, but talk to your physician about other positions depending on your type of arthritis and make sure you do not stress an arthritic joint or pull a painful muscle during sex.

• *Stay on your medications.* Set the timing of your arthritis pain medications so they are fully effective when you are making love. In addition, just as a moist heat is helpful in letting you exercise, a warm bath or shower before sex can soothe painful joints and stiff muscles. Spending time together in a warm Jacuzzi before sex can be romantic and also help you to feel less pain.

• *Be patient.* If you have avoided intimacy because of arthritis pain, allow plenty of time to get your sex life active again. Try to relax and simply enjoy the time; avoid judging it by past experiences. Professionals in sex therapy encourage enjoyment of the moment as the goal—not performance. With openness and an understanding partner, you can find the positions and moments that work best for you without adding further pain or injury to your joints and muscles.

Sleep Tips

Some patients dread bedtime. Not only do they fear restless sleep because of medication side effects, but they are afraid of turning over on a painful joint and causing more joint pain. Many patients say they are not sleepy at bedtime, usually because of inactivity, and spend hours tossing and turning while their bed partner is sound asleep.

One of the most common problems arthritis patients have is getting proper sleep at night, especially in achieving deep level, or stage 4, sleep. Not only does stage 4 sleep allow you to feel alert and energetic and be more productive, it is also vital for restoring your body—repairing tissues

---

Posture Tips

• Standing or walking with your back bent greatly increases the force on the lower back. The best position is standing with your back straight. Perfect posture is not necessary, just good enough to lower the pressure on your back and decrease your arthritis pain.

• Always wear shoes that are comfortable with good support, such as an athletic shoe or work shoe. Higher heels increase the stress on your back. A rubber mat can help cushion your feet and back if you stand or work in one position. When standing, propping one foot on a box or stool for a few minutes may improve comfort.

and skin, building bone and muscle, and strengthening immune function. You might call it "anti-pain" sleep.

Sleep is vital for all people to stay healthy. But for those with arthritis, sound sleep can make the difference between an active day or a day spent in misery, nursing aching joints or muscles. In findings researched by the 2000 National Sleep Foundation (NSF) Sleep in America poll, more than 20 percent of American adults or 42 million people reported that pain or physical discomfort disrupts their sleep a few nights a week or more. It is estimated that more than 75 percent of arthritis patients suffer with sleep-related problems—from restless sleep because of joint pain to sleep arousals associated with flare-ups.

During sleep, your muscles relax, and sensual perceptions are disengaged from the brain (although hearing remains active above a certain threshold). Different hormones interact with the brain, placing a kind of screen between your brain and your consciousness.

Sleep plays a big role in regulating your immune system, and a weakened immune system leaves you vulnerable to illness. You've probably caught a cold or gastrointestinal virus the day after a late night out. That might be because your immune system was in a weakened state from missing quality sleep, making your body easy prey for a virus.

From a host of scientific studies, we know that exposure to viruses and bacteria results in no health problems—if your immune system is strong. Yet when faced with sleep deprivation, the immune system cannot work at full capacity. When your immune system malfunctions, it yields to autoimmune diseases such as some types of arthritis. If your

---

Protect Your Feet

If you suffer from arthritis of the feet, the bones may change position or shape, which can create pressure against the shoe. Your body reacts by forming a callus or corn. Ready-made shoes may not fit the foot in osteoarthritis. Proper shoes may need to be custom made, or surgery may be needed to correct the deformity and allow your usual shoes to fit correctly. Specially made inserts for your shoes can help change the forces on your feet and increase comfort while lowering stress on the joints of the foot.

It would be a wise idea to see a podiatrist to make sure your shoes fit properly and any necessary adjustments are made.

Protect Your Hands

- Make sure that as many joints as possible share the load in any activity you do. This means avoiding favoring a particular finger or position with the hands.
- Seek help with aids and devices. For example, use hook and loop fasteners to replace buttons on clothing. Add accessories to door-knobs for easier turning. Use rotary lamp switches that require just a touch to the lamp base rather than twisting a small knob switch. An extremely convenient tiny tool, the buttonhook, just might take care of all your buttoning problems. Just slip the hook through the buttonhole, catch the button, and pull it back through. A long-handled shoehorn allows you to get your shoes on without bending over as well. Pincer devices, available for hose or socks, elastic-waist pants, and slip-on shoes with elastic laces are also helpful.
- Instead of fumbling for that zipper, try using a zipper ring. It's bigger than the zipper tab on your clothing and gives you more leverage for pulling.
- Cover your knife or other utensil with foam padding or a rubber grip to make the handle larger and require less force on the fingers.
- Use a jar opener and both hands when opening jars to avoid extra force on the hands and finger joints.
- Use lightweight plastic cups and dishes or paper plates and cups instead of heavy china.
- When emptying a heavy food container use a spoon or ladle to remove the contents rather than lifting the heavy container with your hands.
- Use long faucet handles in bathrooms and kitchen to make faucets easier to turn.
- Use foam padding around your pencil or pen. This is available in office supply stores. Put this padding around crochet needles, too, but continue to perform tasks such as crocheting or playing the piano to keep finger joints limber and pliable.
- Use pump toothpastes rather than squeeze tubes.
- Choose lightweight clothing with Velcro closures, or you could add them to clothes.
- Women should use bras that open from the front; men should look for pants that have Velcro closures as opposed to zippers.
- Ponchos that slip over the head and shoulders are preferable over button-up sweaters and jackets.

immune system is depleted, your body can be overwhelmed by bacteria, viruses, or toxicity, which can result in life-threatening diseases.

Some experts now believe that sleep and arthritis pain are related. According to researchers from the University of North Carolina at Chapel Hill, the disruption of sleep appears at times to be a consequence of arthritis pain or even the arthritis medications that many people take. This is a major problem, because people with arthritis pain need more rest and more energy than other people for routine daily tasks. While the study suggests a connection between sleep and arthritis, there may also be a link between exercise and arthritis and a good night's sleep. Here are some pain-free sleep tips.

- *Continue your Exercise Treatment*. Moderate daily exercise is helpful for people with arthritis pain who want to improve their sleep cycle. In findings published in January 1997 in the *Journal of the American Medical Association*, researchers at Stanford University found that moderate-intensity exercise improved quality of sleep in people age fifty-six and seventy-six. Compared to a control group, people who exercised aerobically for 30 to 40 minutes four times per week reported improvement in general quality of sleep, quicker sleep onset, longer sleep duration, and a feeling of being rested in the morning.
- *Take time to rest*. Pain is exhausting, and pain is a leading cause of insomnia. When pain makes it hard to sleep, falling asleep is often the greatest problem. I know that having a chronic disease such as arthritis can make you feel weary. Then, when you add ongoing medications to the pain and illness, is it any wonder you often feel so tired? Daily rest periods can be an easy but important way to reduce pain and increase energy. For instance, I recommend those with very active inflammatory arthritis, such as rheumatoid arthritis or psoriatic arthritis, take a 10-minute short rest period in the late morning and late afternoon. This helps to make the rest of the day better quality and less painful. I have patients who put a cot or couch in their offices and work during this time. Lying down in the company's break room while reading or listening to music can also be energizing.
- *Select a firm mattress for your bed*. If the mattress is too soft, it may put extra stress on your back. Remember that mattresses do not last forever. If your mattress is more than five years old, you may need

Avoiding Computer-Related Back and Neck Pain

Did you know that more than half of all computer users report some type of neck or back pain each year? In a report published in the *American Journal of Industrial Medicine* researchers from Emory University in Atlanta, Georgia, followed 632 men and women who used computers more than fifteen hours a week over a three-year period. The study found that more women than men reported an injury or problem, and one-third of computer users actually develop an impairment or loss of function.

To avoid back or neck pain while working at your computer, use the following strategies:

- Sit properly to reduce the amount of force on your back. The forces are high on the lower back many times each day. For example, sitting with no back support causes 40 percent greater pressure on the lower back than standing. This force increases even more when you sit and lean forward.
- Sitting is less painful and tiring if you use a backrest on your chair at work. Rest your lower back against the back of the chair and use a support for the back to reduce the pressure on the lower spine. This will help to reduce pain and fatigue.
- If you must sit for long periods, stand or walk around your desk for a few minutes every one to two hours. Use a chair with armrests to lower the forces on the back and make sure your feet reach the floor comfortably.
- Make sure your computer chair is comfortable, with arms that can fit under the desk, a firm back support and proper height, so that the feet are comfortably flat on the floor.
- Adjust the height of the level of work to a comfortable position to avoid leaning forward. Remember that sitting in a chair and leaning forward causes higher pressures on the lower spine than sitting straight or standing.
- Make sure that the height of your work desk is comfortable. If it is too high or too low, it adds unnecessary stress to the lower back or neck.
- Stand up and stretch or walk for a few minutes every hour. If this is not possible, try stretching while sitting. (Modify the stretching exercises discussed on page 263 to accommodate your work environment.)
- Purchase wrist rests for your computer desk. Some are made of a comfortable gel structure that lets you reduce stress in the wrist, maintain a neutral comfortable position, and avoid repetitive stress.

to replace it. Some of my patients find the most relief in back pain when they sleep on a waterbed. Each person must find the best mattress for their pain situation, and the optimal recommendation is a mattress that it not too soft, not too hard, and allows good, restful sleep.

• *Get an orthopedic pillow.* There are many types of orthopedic pillows that can give different parts of your body excellent support. For instance, some fit the contour of the neck or back. Others support the hips or knees. Use the websites in the Resources section at the end of the book, and search for the pillows that work best for your type of arthritis.

• *Sleep on your stomach.* If you have arthritis in your back, you might find it helpful to spend time sleeping on your stomach. This may also help with posture, especially in helping to prevent the stooped-over stance. In ankylosing spondylitis, for example, sleeping on the stomach for 30 minutes each night can help prevent deformity in the back.

• *Use an electric blanket during winter months.* Some arthritis patients report great pain when heavy quilts or blankets touch their painful joints. You can resolve this problem by relying on a quality electric blanket on cold nights. Find one that is lightweight and that provides ample heat. A thermal blanket can also produce light-weight warmth.

• *Use mind-body exercises to relax at bedtime.* High levels of arousal associated with racing thoughts, worrying, or rumination may also delay sleep onset, or worries may cause you to have restless sleep or to wake up early. Meditation or guided imagery (see Step 6) can help you relax at night as you learn to focus your thoughts on a neutral or enjoyable target.

• *Avoid alcohol before bedtime.* A nightcap may make you sleepy at first, but you'll sleep less soundly and wake up more tired as a result. Alcohol and other depressants suppress Rapid Eye Movement (REM) sleep, the time in which most dreaming occurs. Less REM sleep is associated with more night awakenings and a more restless sleep. If you drink alcohol at night, be aware of the amount and whether your sleep is more fragmented and broken after drinking. If so, avoid alcohol so you can get the six to eight hours of uninterrupted sleep needed to feel refreshed.

• *Use the bedroom for sleep and sex only.* The TV should be in another room since it stimulates the brain and arouses the nervous system.

Let's Review: 8 Steps to Making Key Lifestyle Changes

1. Review the lifestyle changes in this step, and then take notes in your Pain-Free Diary of those that may help your situation.
2. Take a walk through your home—both inside and outside—and write down areas that need attention. Designate an hour one Saturday to make a fall-proof home.
3. Evaluate your daily calendar and schedule. Follow the suggestions to ease stress by pacing yourself, organizing your life, and delegating responsibilities to those around you.
4. Consider taking up gardening as a hobby and as exercise. Bending, stooping, raking, and digging all help to work your joints and muscles, and the end product—healthy plants—is an added bonus.
5. Plan to travel in the next few months. Follow the tips on traveling with arthritis and your trip should be pain-free. Talk to your doctor ahead of time for additional advice, and make sure you have ample medications. You might ask your local support group about special trips or cruises for those with this disease.
6. Rest and sleep are crucial for a pain-free life. Evaluate your bedroom to make sure it is suitable for a good night's sleep. If you are noise sensitive, get earplugs at your local pharmacy. If light causes you to awaken frequently, buy a sleep mask at any department store.
7. There are plenty of ways to be intimate with your partner, even with arthritis. Talk openly with your partner, using the discussion in this step, and together discover new ways to find sexual pleasure.
8. Protect your joints. No matter which joint is affected with arthritis, you can protect them in your daily activities. Follow the Pain-Free Program instructions and make sure your joints are treated royally.

Make family decisions and argue, if necessary, in a common family area, and avoid any major decision before bedtime.

- *Keep the temperature cool—about 67 degrees F (19 degrees C).* Cool air helps to naturally lower your body temperature and slow the metabolism, both necessary to achieve a very dormant physical state. A warm bath before bedtime may help to increase the chance of falling into a sound sleep.
- *Make sure the bedroom is quiet.* Wear earplugs if noises disturb you while sleeping. Some people find that it helps to hear "white noise" from a machine that produces a humming sound or by turning the radio to a station that has gone off the air.

How Pain and Poor Sleep Disturb Your Life

General Mood and Disposition	Ability to Handle Daily Stress
Physical Health	Ability to Concentrate
Emotional Health	Productivity
Mental Health	Ability to Motivate for Daily Tasks

Doctor's Pain-Free Treatment

Osteoarthritis

- Review the strategies for creating a fall-proof home and make sure your home follows this plan.
- Check out the Resources section at the end of the book to find assistive devices for daily living tasks that will ease the workload on your joints.
- Make sure your desk or computer chair has a high back and armrests. Check to see if your feet touch the floor to take pressure off the spine.

Fibromyalgia

- Take note of ways to alleviate additional stress in your life using POD. Pay particular attention to Organize—getting rid of those commitments that are unnecessary, *Additional Tasks*, so you can focus on *Essential Tasks*.
- Make sure you allow daily times for rest and exercise as you use POD.
- Find ways to enjoy gardening, travel, and intimacy even with your fibromyalgia symptoms. Sometimes a return to normal activities can boost mood and increase sound sleep.

Carpal Tunnel Syndrome

- Find ways to avoid overuse of your wrist, using the suggestions on page 107.
- Always support your injured wrist with the other wrist when lifting heavy objects.

Bursitis and Tendonitis

- Review ways to protect your joints from further injury. See if these suggestions may help you avoid getting bursitis or tendonitis again.
- Fall-proof your home to avoid further injury.

Rheumatoid Arthritis (and Other Inflammatory Types)
- Review the fall-proof steps and make sure your home is safe. Pay special attention to areas where you could trip to avoid injuring painful, arthritic joints.
- Follow the suggestions in POD and learn to pace yourself. By accepting your limitations and allowing for rest times and periodic time-outs, you will increase energy, alertness, and your ability to be productive—without pain.
- Find strategies to prevent further injury to joints and follow these tips.
- Do not let your arthritis keep you from living a full life. Read the suggestions on gardening, travel, intimacy, and sleep, and ask your doctor for more information on how you can return to normal daily activities.

Consider Bodywork and Massage

When forty-seven-year-old Judith came to our clinic two years ago, her husband pushed her in a wheelchair because of intense pain in her right knee. This once-active mother of four was about forty pounds overweight and could barely walk because of pain and stiffness.

After ordering some tests, including X rays, I told Judith she had osteoarthritis, a common "wear and tear" type of arthritis that affects millions of Americans. I prescribed a nonsteroidal anti-inflammatory drug (NSAID) for pain and stiffness, along with resistance exercises to build strength in the muscles supporting the knee and regular applications of moist heat to reduce inflammation.

Judith agreed to follow this basic treatment plan for osteoarthritis and also said she'd try modifying her diet to help her lose weight. After she left that day, I didn't see her again, until a year later when she stopped by to tell me her knee pain had completely resolved. Judith had lost nearly thirty-five pounds, which she attributed to a healthier diet and daily exercise on her stationary bike, and she was seeing a licensed massage therapist each week. She said the therapist performed deep muscle massage on her leg and her lower back and wrapped her knee in warm, moist towels for about 15 minutes each session to help reduce pain and increase mobility.

As a physician, I know losing weight gave Judith great relief of pain and allowed her to be more active. Particularly for osteoarthritis of the knee, weight loss is a key factor in pain relief. In addition, the biking exercise helped to build muscle strength and kept her arthritic knee flexible. Yet, I am also a believer in massage and other touch therapies as a complement

---

Gather Your Pain-Free Tools

1. In your Pain-Free Diary record the particular massage or bodywork modalities that appeal to you. Talk to your doctor about these therapies and see if they are safe for your situation.
2. Make an appointment with a licensed massage therapist to have a gentle massage. Record your feelings in your Pain-Free Diary after having this touch therapy. If your pain was reduced, consider having another massage in a week or two.
3. If you have health insurance, check with your insurance provider to see if massage therapy is covered. Many companies now include alternative therapies, such as massage, as part of their integrative medicine coverage.

---

to traditional methods in helping to ease the pain of arthritis. I commended Judith in taking control of her arthritis and living pain-free.

Complement Your Pain-Free Program

By now, you should be getting a good idea of what it takes to live pain-free—even with a chronic disease like arthritis. In Step 1, I explained how exercise and moist heat could reduce inflammation and keep joints healthy and muscles strong. The Pain-Free Nutritional Plan discussed in Step 2 can help you to maintain a normal weight—key for easing pain on weight-bearing joints. Trying some alternative therapies such as glucosamine for osteoarthritis or herbal remedies like valerian to help induce sleep may let you cut back on medications. In addition, making key lifestyle changes, as outlined in Step 4, can make all the difference in your comfort at home and at work.

Many of my patients depend on massage, structural alignment, chiropractic, or acupuncture for additional pain relief or stress reduction. In this step, I want to discuss the benefits of complementing your Pain-Free Program with massage therapy or manual manipulation to ease arthritis pain and stiffness. I will also describe specific tools, such as electrical stimulation and ultrasound, that are often used in conjunction with manual manipulation treatments. I will outline the most useful therapies, and then make recommendations for your particular type of arthritis.

First, let me tell you about one of my patient's positive experiences with healing touch.

Kristin, a forty-two-year-old freelance journalist, has had rheumatoid arthritis for almost a decade and found massage to be extremely effective as a complement to her pain management program. "A few years ago, I asked my primary care doctor about bodywork and whether it might help ease my body aches and stiffness. He shrugged and said there was not much science to back up bodywork for arthritis pain. However, I was sick and tired of feeling sick and tired, and I decided to try touch therapy anyway.

"When I went to the appointment at a nearby massage therapy center, I was impressed at how professional everyone was. The receptionist asked me to fill out a medical history form, and then one of the therapists took me in a room to give me some background. I didn't realize the therapists were licensed after taking a two-year program and undergoing twenty-two hundred hours of practical training.

"The therapist showed me to a dressing area where I exchanged my street clothes for a long white sheet, which I discreetly tucked around my body. I then sat on the long table, and the therapist began to rub sweet-smelling sesame oil on my skin, as she softly kneaded my tight muscles. Using a gentle, rocking motion, she helped to release tension out of my upper body, and then had me lie down facing the table. Her hands worked up and down my back. Sometimes I felt like her fingers were pointing right into my skin, but she said that's where my muscles were so tense. She focused mostly on my upper body—my neck, shoulders, and upper back—where my arthritis pain was the worst.

"After the massage, I was almost afraid to move. I was incredibly relaxed and the pain was almost nonexistent. Finally, as I was getting dressed, I realized that the range of motion in both of my arms was greater and the tension in my upper body was greatly reduced. I continued receiving thirty-minute weekly massages for six months and had greatly reduced pain and stiffness, less fatigue, and less difficulty sleeping. While my primary care doctor gave me the accurate diagnosis, it was hands-on touch that gave me a normal life again."

Massage

Technically speaking, bodywork is the umbrella term that refers to the hands-on techniques to treat problems that usually occur with the musculoskeletal system and to promote relaxation within the body. The basic philosophy of massage therapy is to help the body to heal itself, and in doing so, it will increase health and well-being.

How it Works
Massage involves the manipulation of soft tissues with the hands through rubbing, stroking, pressure, and so on. Swedish massage is probably the most commonly used hands-on therapy to help ease arthritis pain, particularly to ease back and neck pain, muscle pain, and stress.

Step Back in Time
Massage and manipulation to ease pain are not New Age therapies for arthritis. More than two thousand years ago, the ancient Greek physician Hippocrates wrote that doctors should be experienced in "rubbing that can bind a joint that is loose and loosen a joint that is too hard." In Egypt, there is the tomb of Ankh-Mahor from 2200 B.C., known as the Tomb of the Physician. In one of the wall pictures, two men are having their extremities treated with massage. According to documents, the Roman naturalist Pliny was rubbed to ease his asthma, and Julius Caesar was pinched all over daily to ease headaches and neuralgia.

Massage was not a prominent medical therapy until the early nineteenth century when people such as Per Henrik Ling, a physiologist, fencing master, and gymnast, began to study this alternative therapy. Ling suffered from chronic and painful arthritis and was determined to find a cure. Tagged the Father of Modern Massage, Ling even traveled to China to learn the various techniques to cure his rheumatism. On his return, Ling developed a system of medical gymnastics known as the Swedish Movement Cure. These techniques included *effleurage*, *petrissage* or pressing and squeezing, and *tapotement*. His system of massage was later integrated into Swedish massage.

Pain-Free Benefits
Massage is helpful for increasing circulation of blood to tense, sore muscles. It may be used in conjunction with ultrasound (see page 125) or with the application of heat or cold. Massage is also helpful for removing built-up toxins such as lactic acid and helps re-educate muscles and joints that have become misaligned.

Massage boosts the hormone oxytocin, which promotes feelings of well-being and calmness. Oxytocin is the hormone best known for its role in inducing labor and is tagged the "quintessential maternal hormone."

When it is released into the brain, it is known to promote calming and positive social behaviors. In humans, oxytocin is released during sexual orgasm in both men and women. Yet some newer studies show that increased levels of oxytocin can reduce levels of the stress hormone cortisol, ease anxiety, and positively affect relationships.

In a revealing study published in 1999 in the journal *Psychiatry*, researchers measured oxytocin levels in twenty-five women and found that blood levels of the hormone oxytocin rose significantly following neck and shoulder massages. Because chronic elevation of the stress hormone cortisol is a predictor for early onset of hypertension and other chronic diseases, reducing cortisol may help you live longer and feel healthier.

Massage may block pain signals to the brain with a process called the gate control theory. First proposed in 1965, the gate control theory suggests that there is a "gating system" in the central nervous system that opens and closes to let pain messages to the brain or block them. The basis for the theory is the belief that psychological as well as physical factors channel the brain's understanding of painful feelings and the ensuing response. When you massage your skin, this sends other impulses along the same nerves. When all these impulses try to reach the brain through nerves, the nerves get congested, and most impulses do not reach the brain. Massage or touch therapies work by "closing the gate" that pain impulses have to pass through.

Massage helps to improve joint movement, relax tense muscles, and stimulate the flow of blood and nutrients to the skin and underlying tissues. What's more, these hands-on therapies are useful for painful conditions as a means to break the pain cycle and increase tolerance of exercise. A study published in May 2002 in the journal *Annals of Internal Medicine* confirmed that manual therapy performed by chiropractors, osteopaths, and physical and massage therapists was the best choice in improving neck mobility and reducing pain. Another study, published in the April 2001 issue of the journal *Archives of Internal Medicine*, revealed that patients who used regular massage for back pain had the least costs for medication and health care.

Massage aids in relaxation and stress reduction. In a study conducted by Tiffany Field, Ph.D., and colleagues, children with mild to moderate juvenile rheumatoid arthritis were massaged by their parents 15 minutes a day for thirty days while a control group received relaxation therapies. Researchers reported that immediately after massage, the children's anxiety and stress hormone (cortisol) levels were decreased. In findings

Techniques

- Effleurage—Long, gliding str
- Petrissage—Pressure applied a
- Friction—Deep massage appli
  or fingertips
- Kneading—Squeezing across th
- Hacking—Light slaps or karate

Pain

published in 1997 in th
said the assessment

120

Types of Bo
Swedish N
ing, an
mu

Try Self-Massage

You don't have to get a professional massage to benefit from touch therapy. If you have tension in your neck, shoulders, wrists, or elsewhere, you can massage these areas gently with your fingers to ease tight muscles and decrease stiffness.

1. Use a few drops of a massage oil in your hand, and gently touch the back of your neck, gently rubbing the oil into the skin.
2. As you make contact with the skin, start using a circular motion with your fingertips, gently moving up and down the neck.
3. Work outward down the side of the neck to your shoulders, continuing the gentle circular motion.
4. Squeeze your shoulders with your hand, one at a time, using the opposite hand. Then, using long, stroking motions, gently sweep the skin from the neck to the shoulder and down to the elbow.

Who Seeks Massage Therapy?

Today, there are more than a quarter-million massage therapists in the United States, and nearly one-fifth of American adults claim to get a professional massage each year. It may surprise you that of all the age groups, those who are most likely to seek massage are the baby boomers, according to a survey taken by Oxford Health Plans. When offered, 100 percent of workers age 45 to 54 took advantage of a massage, against 60 percent of workers age 18 to 34; 20 percent of workers age 35 to 44; and 50 percent of workers age 55 and older.

Journal of Pediatric Psychology researchers also
pain was decreased over the thirty-day period.

ork and Massage

ssage. Swedish massage uses a system of long strokes, knead-
friction techniques to massage the more superficial layers of the
les. This hands-on touch is combined with active and passive move-
ents of the joints. The practitioner may use aromatic oil on the skin to
help facilitate the stroking and kneading of the body, thereby stimulating
metabolism and circulation. The therapist applies pressure and rubs the
muscles in the same direction as the flow of blood returning to the heart.
Swedish massage is said to help flush the tissues of lactic and uric acids,
as well as to improve circulation without increasing the load on the heart.

Make sure you choose a registered massage therapist who holds the
appropriate diploma, certificate, or equivalent from an accredited
massage therapy school. Many states regulate massage therapists and
require five hundred hours of instruction before being offered a license.

Trager Work. Trager work involves gentle, hands-on manipulation of
the limbs, joints, and muscles in an effort to train the mind in body
awareness. This type of bodywork is based on the theory that body
tension results in pain and stems from trauma, weak posture, fear,
emotional blockages, and/or stress. The practitioner's goal is to help you
unconsciously realize that movement is effortless and without pain.

There are two parts to the complete Trager approach. First, the
practitioner uses tablework (work on a special table), which involves
rhythmic hands-on therapies such as rocking, stretching, and loosening
tight muscles and painful joints. Once you are relaxed, the Trager practitioner gives instruction in movements (Mentastics, or mental gymnastics)
that will help to alleviate tension, tight muscles, and increase mobility.

Make sure the practitioner you choose has completed more than 250
hours of training and is certified by the Trager Institute. (If you have
rheumatoid arthritis, talk to your arthritis specialist before doing Trager.)

Polarity Therapy. Polarity therapy uses gentle touch and stretching exercises with the intent of establishing a balanced flow of energy in the body,
thus helping it to heal. Combining therapies from Western and Eastern
medicine, the practitioner will mix bodywork, nutritional counseling, yoga,
counseling, and acupressure to balance the body's energy.

Although there is no licensing for polarity therapists, qualified persons
should have completed 155 hours of coursework to practice as an

associate practitioner and 460 additional hours to be a registered polarity practitioner. These guidelines are set by the American Polarity Therapy Association (APTA). Ask your doctor or chiropractor for a referral.

Feldenkrais Method. Feldenkrais method combines gentle movement therapy and hands-on massage that can help increase range of motion and improve breathing. This therapy is based on the theory that the central nervous system plays an important role in how we feel. Using the Feldenkrais method, you become fully aware of your skeleton, muscles, and joints, and also become more conscious of negative posture and movements. Correcting the poor posture or how you hold your body can often alleviate unnecessary pain.

Trainers undergo 800 to 1,000 hours of instruction over a four-year period. Make sure your practitioner is certified by the Feldenkrais Guild of North America, the professional association for the discipline, in Albany, Oregon.

Hellerwork. Hellerwork entails movement education and deep tissue massage that helps to realign the body and reduce chronic arthritis pain. This touch therapy is based on the theory that your body can get out of alignment because of stress, which can cause the tissue (connective tissue that encases the muscle and connects muscle to bone) to become taut and inflexible. Using pressure and stroking, practitioners work to elongate or stretch the tightened fascia to make it more flexible. As the fascia becomes softer, the body restores back to its natural balance.

The specialist you choose should be a certified Hellerwork practitioner who has undergone 1,250 hours of study and training. (If you are pregnant or have rheumatoid arthritis, talk to your doctor before doing Hellerwork.)

Rolfing/Structural Integration. Rolfing is a system of body restructuring and movement that focuses on the connective tissue that surrounds muscles, to release tension. The Rolfer manipulates the fascia instead of the muscles (as with other types of bodywork). Using the knuckles, fingers, elbows, and knees, the practitioner manipulates the fascia to release tension and stress.

Try to find a practitioner who has at least a basic training certificate in Rolfing, which takes from one to two years.

Aston-Patterning. An offshoot of Rolfing, Aston-Patterning is a form of muscle manipulation that combines exercises with a gentler form of Rolfing and targets chronic muscle problems. The practitioner looks for muscle tightness and structural formation, then uses a combination of massage and education techniques to help the client retrain their muscles. Using a special "spiraling" technique, the therapist will work to relax the muscles and loosen tight joints, permitting the body to revert to a healthier posture. Aston-Patterning therapists teach special fitness exercises to help keep muscle patterns healthy as well as make environmental suggestions, such as changing the height of your computer chair or armrest supports to keep the spine aligned.

Choose a bodywork specialist (physical or occupational therapist or nurse practitioner) who is a certified graduate of the Aston Training Center in Nevada.

Myotherapy. Myotherapy uses applied pressure and stretching on trigger points (tender spots in the muscle or other soft tissue) to relieve tension and pain. This therapy is especially helpful for those with fibromyalgia since the practitioner uses fingers, knuckles, or elbows to work directly on the knots in muscles, giving greater mobility without pain.

Choose a practitioner who is highly knowledgeable in the area of kinesiology, which is the study of human structure and function and its relationship to health and movement. In some states, myotherapists must also be licensed massage therapists.

Choosing a Practitioner and Therapy

Just like you interview a doctor, it's important to interview a massage or bodywork practitioner ahead of time to make sure this person is the right professional to serve you. Some questions to ask include the following:

- What are your credentials? Are you licensed?
- Where did you do your training? How many hours did you study?
- Do you have any clients I could ask for references?
- What will the treatment involve?
- How long will I need the treatment?
- What are the advantages and disadvantages of this therapy as opposed to other alternatives? Can I use the treatment along with my regular conventional medical therapy?
- Is this treatment safe? Are there studies to support it?
- How much will each session cost?
- Does insurance cover the cost?
- When should I see results?
- Are there any dangerous side effects I should be aware of?
- Can my doctor call you regarding the treatment to keep communication open?

Chiropractic

Chiropractic, the largest alternative medicine profession, is another popular hands-on therapy that has given millions of arthritis patients relief, particularly those with back pain or shoulder pain. Founded in the late 1800s, this therapy focuses on restoring proper balance and structure to the spine and joints with the goal of restoring healthy function to the nervous system.

How it Works

To resolve symptoms, the doctor of chiropractic focuses on adjusting the spine with a specific directional thrust. The doctor administers the adjustment or a specific force in a precise direction applied to the joint that is fixated, locked up, or not moving properly.

Doctors of chiropractic base their practice on the theory that the nervous system controls all functions in the body. Messages must travel from your brain down your spinal cord, then out to the nerves at particular parts of the body, and then back to the spinal cord and up to the brain. The theory is that abnormal positions of the spinal bones may interfere with these messages and are often the underlying cause of many health problems.

Pain-Free Benefits

Chiropractic is successfully used to treat back or neck pain, and pain from musculoskeletal injuries. Many patients with fibromyalgia find that this alternative hands-on therapy improves pain levels and increases cervical and lumbar ranges of motion.

Spinal manipulation (or adjustment) attempts to relieve pain by increasing the mobility between spinal vertebrae that have become restricted or out of position. By applying specific procedures by hand, the chiropractic practitioner attempts to restore mobility to the joints to allow a more normal and natural position. The manipulations may be gentle stretching or pressure maneuvers, multiple repeated motions in the same area, or specific high-velocity thrusts to treat the joints. You may feel a stretching or popping sensation with the treatments. The chiropractor may recommend a series of treatments until maximum relief is felt. It is hoped that the treatments improve mobility, reduce inflammation and nerve irritation, as well as reduce muscle spasm and pain. Just after the treatments there may be a temporary increase in back or neck pain, or there may be immediate relief of pain.

Alert

A chiropractor is not a medical doctor, so it's important to work with your doctor for an accurate diagnosis and other specific medical treatment. Make sure you know which type of arthritis you have (osteoarthritis or inflammatory arthritis), since the treatment may vary, depending on this diagnosis. Your chiropractor will not typically treat with manipulation if there is any concern about possible fracture, infection, cancer, or some types of severe arthritis. Your medical doctor can work together with your chiropractic physician.

Along with the adjustments and manipulation, the chiropractor may also recommend a program of rehabilitation to stabilize and reduce joint involvement, rehabilitate muscle ligament tissue, and balance nerve impulses. Many chiropractic clinics provide diet counseling and stress reduction techniques.

Physical Therapy

Your doctor may recommend that you see a physical therapist to organize and plan your exercise program. Physical therapists are also trained and certified in the use of many treatments such as acupuncture or ultrasound, which can help the pain, stiffness, and swelling of arthritis. These methods can help build muscle strength, which gives more support and flexibility to your joints. Your physical therapist will evaluate your condition and, with your doctor, can plan the best combination of moist heat and exercises for your own situation. Your therapist may use a combination of whirlpool, heated pool, moist heating pads or packs, ultrasound, ice, and at times other methods, such as acupuncture or electrical stimulation, to help decrease pain and inflammation.

Your physical therapist will also help design an exercise program that starts slowly and gradually but will achieve your goals of increased muscle strength and joint motion. At first, this may be manually moving your joints throughout their range of motion if they are painful. As your pain improves, exercise is done with more and more of your own active effort until you can do the exercises entirely on your own.

The physical therapist will tailor a program for your individual needs so that when you finish your sessions after a few weeks you will understand how to continue an effective program at home. Using the follow-up program at home, over the months you will continue your improvement to the level you want to achieve. Once you begin to feel the results of this exercise program, the longer you continue, the more improvement you'll see.

Occupational Therapy

Physical therapy departments usually include health care professionals educated in occupational therapy. This health professional is trained and certified in evaluating and adapting daily activities for arthritis and other problems. Occupational therapists are trained in the proper construction and demonstration of the use of splints for problems such as arthritis in the hands and wrists and carpal tunnel syndrome; splints protect the joints while at rest or allow activity while still protecting the joints.

Your occupational therapist can show you how to perform many daily tasks in ways that allow you to be more active with the least amount of pain while still protecting your joints. For example, simple devices such as jar openers can greatly lower pressure on your hands and wrists. Canes and other devices, discussed in Step 4, can help you walk more comfortably and safely. Toilet seat extensions make it less work (and less painful) to arise from the toilet. Specially designed or adapted pens, pencils, forks, and other utensils are easily obtained to make your joints less painful and more effective.

Transcutaneous Electrical Nerve Stimulation (TENS)

The physical therapist may use transcutaneous electrical nerve stimulation (TENS) to help alleviate your pain. The gate control theory (page 118) explains the principle behind TENS. With TENS, electrical impulses are sent to certain nerves that block the messages of pain being sent by other nerves from the painful area. These impulses might also cause the body to release endorphins, which are natural pain relievers produced by the body.

It's estimated that from 10 to 35 percent of patients with chronic back pain may have increased relief from this therapy. One of the benefits of TENS is that you can receive instruction on how to use this at home for acute pain flares.

Ultrasound

The physical therapist may use ultrasound to alleviate pain. Ultrasound is a form of deep heating in which sound waves delivered at a frequency above the human range of hearing are applied to the skin and penetrate into the soft tissues, muscles, and tendons. This may help decrease inflammation and improve pain of tender points around painful joints and muscles. The improvement in pain may allow you to perform more exercises that are effective in reducing inflammation.

Traditional Chinese Medicine Therapies

Chinese medicine has become more appealing to Americans, especially with its focus on balance, harmony, and self-care. This ancient medicine is as old as the Chinese civilization itself and gets its theoretical basis from the Taoist principles of yin and yang, the five movements, and *qi* (pronounced "chi"). According to Chinese philosophy, when the body is in balance between yin and yang, health is predominant. Yet when the yin and yang are imbalanced, disease occurs.

Chinese medicine practitioners view yin and yang as a way of seeing life, in which all things work together to be part of a whole; nothing is seen in isolation or as absolute. This philosophy of healing is contrary to Western medicine where a specific disease may be treated separately without considering the total health of the person—mind, body, and spirit.

In Oriental medicine, *qi* is the life force of all living things and represents all energy within the universe. In the body, *qi* travels among twelve imaginary meridians (also called pathways or channels) to keep the body nourished. These meridians start at your fingertips, connect to the brain, and then connect to the organ associated with the specific meridian. The twelve major meridians correspond to specific human organs: kidneys, liver, spleen, heart, lungs, pericardium, bladder, gallbladder, stomach, small and large intestines, and the triple burner (body temperature regulator).

Traditional Chinese Medicine practitioners believe that when *qi* is blocked or thrown off balance, illness or symptoms result. Both rheumatoid arthritis and osteoarthritis are known as *bi* (or blockage) syndromes. If you have deep muscle or joint pain, the Traditional Chinese Medicine explanation is that the channel running through that site has been physically disrupted, resulting in local pain. To treat this, practitioners locate the point in the body where *qi* is blocked and restore the flow of energy using acupuncture, acupressure, or other therapies.

Acupuncture
Acupuncture has a long history in Traditional Chinese Medicine. Although more than three hundred acupuncture points have been

described in Chinese literature, only about a hundred are used by practitioners in the West. When the practitioner touches one of these points, the point refers to healing another part of the body. For example, a point on your second toe is used to treat headaches and toothaches; a point near your elbow helps to boost immune function. Charts are available showing the exact points and the corresponding benefit in the body.

How Acupuncture Works

To receive the treatment, you will lie down on a table or sit in a chair so that the practitioner has access to the skin at specific points. When the tiny needle is inserted into one point on the body, it stimulates nerves in the underlying muscles. This stimulation sends impulses up the spinal cord to the limbic system, a primitive part of the brain. The impulses also go to the midbrain and the pituitary gland. Studies show that acupuncture may alter brain chemistry by changing the way neurotransmitters, biochemical substances that stimulate or inhibit nerve impulses in the brain, relay information about external stimuli and sensations, such as pain. Acupuncture also has been documented to affect the parts of the central nervous system related to sensation and involuntary body functions, such as immune reactions and processes whereby your blood pressure, blood flow, and body temperature are regulated.

The acupuncture needles are left in place from a few seconds up to one hour, depending on how the practitioner wants to influence the flow of *qi* in the body. Sometimes moxibustion is used to warm the body's *qi* before inserting the needles. This involves a centuries-old process of heating special herbs and holding them above the acupoint.

Electro-acupuncture uses stimulation of specific trigger points on the body with small electrical impulses (milliamp/microamp) through acupuncture needles or with electro-stim handheld cutaneous probes.

Pain-Free Benefits

Acupuncture may help to relieve some types of arthritis pain, particularly fibromyalgia and osteoarthritis. One particular study, conducted at the University of Maryland School of Medicine, compared acupuncture to conventional medical care for osteoarthritis. The participants who had received acupuncture showed improvements at four and at eight weeks, although those improvements tended to decline after twelve weeks.

In a study published in the April 2001 issue of *Arthritis and Rheumatism*, researchers found that acupuncture gave excellent pain relief to those with osteoarthritis in the knees—relief that was not qualified as placebo. The National Institute of Health concluded that acupuncture could be useful as an additional treatment, as an alternative, or as part of a comprehensive management program for fibromyalgia.

Still more evidence in acupuncture's favor was reported at the 2001 Annual Meeting of the American College of Rheumatology, as researchers gave findings that acupuncture helps relieve symptoms such as pain and depression in women with fibromyalgia. Symptoms continued to lessen over a period of time.

Acupressure

Using gentle pressure, this hands-on therapy is applied with the thumb or index finger at specific "trigger points" on the body. Traditional Chinese Medicine practitioners believe that by stimulating these trigger points, it releases energy or unblocks *qi*, resulting in health and healing.

How Acupressure Works

During treatment, each point is held with a steady pressure for one to three minutes, using the tips or balls of the fingers or thumb. If the acupressure point is sensitive or tender, this indicates that the meridian (energy pathway or channel) is blocked. During the treatment, this tenderness should dissipate as the channel becomes unblocked and energy flows freely again.

Pain-Free Benefits

On the physical level, acupressure affects muscular tension, blood circulation, and other physiological parameters. On a scientific level, researchers find that both acupressure and acupuncture cause the body to release endorphins and monoamines, chemicals that block pain signals in the spinal cord and the brain. The endorphin system consists of chemicals that regulate the activity of a group of nerve cells in the brain that relax muscles, dull pain, and reduce panic and anxiety. The system can also lower blood pressure and reduce the heart's workload. These ancient touch therapies may also trigger the release of more hormones, including serotonin, a brain chemical that makes you feel calm and serene, as well as the anti-inflammatory chemical known as cortisol. With acupressure, not only are you benefiting from stimulating the trigger points, but also from increased circulation and decreased tension.

Shiatsu

Originating in China about two thousand years ago, shiatsu is a combination of *anma* (Chinese massage) and acupuncture. This healing therapy was adopted by the Japanese for aches, pains, and chronic illness. Shiatsu, as we know it today, was founded about a hundred years ago, and there are now more than 87,000 certified shiatsu practitioners in Japan.

Shiatsu draws on the notion of *qi*, and the sessions focus on relieving pain and helping the body rid itself of any toxins before they develop into illness.

How Shiatsu Works

The shiatsu practitioner applies gentle to deep pressure to specific points (*tsubos*) on the meridians. Practitioners may apply pressure to the *tsubos*

Let's Review: 8 Steps to Getting Started with Bodywork and Massage

1. Talk to your doctor to make sure hands-on therapies will help in your situation. Continue to do the twice-daily moist heat applications or baths, and take your prescribed medications for optimal pain relief.
2. Use the criteria on page 122 to assess a massage therapist before undergoing treatment. Make sure the person you choose is licensed in the field or has excellent credentials.
3. Review the steps on page 119 and learn how to use self-massage on arthritic joints to alleviate stiffness and pain.
4. If you find relief, a periodic evaluation and treatment by a physician skilled in chiropractic manipulation may be a part of the overall pain program for arthritis.
5. Ask your doctor if physical therapy might help your arthritis condition. Be sure the physical therapist and your physician discuss your arthritis problem before your visit so the program is specifically designed to meet your arthritis and other health needs.
6. Ask your doctor or physical therapist to demonstrate how TENS is used and see if this might help your pain level between visits.
7. Acupressure is a touch therapy that can be done at any time. Talk to a certified practitioner to learn how to massage acupoints that correspond to your joint or muscle pain.
8. Continue with Steps 1 to 4 as you add massage and bodywork to the Pain-Free Program to ease muscle aches and joint pain and to help increase joint motion.

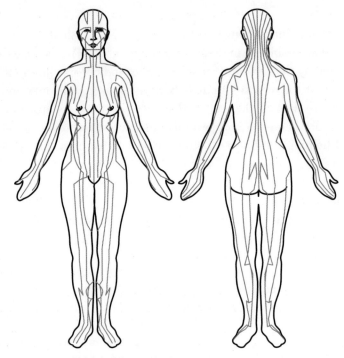

Figure 5.1.

Meridians and acupoints in the body. Each of the twelve organs is linked with a meridian or channel of energy, named according to the internal organ it affects.

using their palms, fingers, elbows, knees, and feet, but work mostly with their thumbs held side by side. For more concentrated pressure, the thumbs are placed on top of one another. Generally, the pressure is held for several seconds and is repeated several times before the practitioner moves to another *tsubo*.

Pain-Free Benefits

The shiatsu pressure may stimulate the body's endorphins to produce a tranquilizing effect. Because shiatsu involves stretching and light manipulation, it helps to loosen muscles and improve blood circulation.

Hands-On Therapies Are Therapeutic

Last year during a regular visit to a nearby retirement village, I stopped to check on my patient Anna. This eighty-nine-year-old woman has osteoarthritis in most of her joints, and when her pain flares up, she prefers to keep to herself.

This particular day, as I rubbed my hand over Anna's arthritic wrist, I couldn't help but notice a faint smile appear on her face. Knowing her history, I don't think the manipulation of her tiny bones did anything magical to alleviate the ravages of her pain. However, being in a nursing home, I know Anna was devoid of human touch, except for the nurse feeling her pulse upon awakening each day. As I gently rubbed her tiny wrist, I could sense her feeling of relief that someone cared.

When I returned to the nursing home the next week, Anna was sitting on the couch in the TV lounge with two friends. All three women reached out to me with their frail, arthritic wrists, longing for the healing power of human touch!

Of all the alternative therapies I recommend, I can always count on massage or hands-on therapies to give comfort. Many believe that if there isn't strong scientific substantiation, then a therapy is not valid. I disagree. I believe that if a treatment works and causes no harm—whether conventional or alternative—then it should be considered. In that regard, hands-on therapies such as massage and bodywork may complement your Pain-Free Program and help you to live an active life again.

Doctor's Pain-Free Treatment

Osteoarthritis
- Try massage to ease sore muscles, especially in the back and neck.
- Chiropractic manipulation might help reduce pain, especially in the back and neck.
- A physical therapist can make sure you're doing the best strengthening exercises for your arthritis, whether it is in your knees, hips, back, shoulders, hands, or other areas. After physical therapy, you should be able to continue the exercise program on your own.

Fibromyalgia
- Regular deep-muscle massage might be effective for alleviating pain trigger points and muscle pain.
- Chiropractic treatment may help ease neck and back pain.
- A physical therapist can guide you in learning the proper technique to stretching and strengthening, as well as help you establish a beginning conditioning program.

Carpal Tunnel Syndrome
- An occupational therapist can show you how to use wrist splints to relieve pain and numbness.
- Check out acupuncture for carpal tunnel syndrome. Be sure to choose an experienced practitioner who is licensed.

Bursitis/Tendonitis
- A physical therapist can help you learn the correct exercises to increase flexibility and strength and prevent future attacks.

Rheumatoid Arthritis (and Other Inflammatory Arthritis)
- Consider regular massage therapy, especially if you have sore muscle pain and limited movement.
- A physical therapist can ensure correct motion and strengthening exercises from the start. Once you've learned the proper form and motion, you can continue the Exercise Treatment at home.
- An occupational therapist can help if your arthritis is severe or you have trouble with daily tasks. You can learn tips on joint protection and try new products that help make daily living tasks easier.

Tap in to Pain-Free Mind Power

It's no news that arthritis is a great source of stress in your life. Whether from the pain itself or the unending limitations in activity, loss of work, and high cost of treatment, arthritis is a chronic stressor. After months of arthritis pain, most patients experience anxiety, irritability, and negative thinking. As the illness and chronic pain cause more stress, they become depressed and are unable to handle the daily functions of life. Painful arthritis flare-ups cause the stress to soar, making it difficult to cope with life's everyday interruptions. This cycle of pain can render you incapable of functioning at home or work and easily interferes with any relationship. Chronic arthritis pain can cause disabling symptoms, including interrupted sleep, muscle spasms, and depression—all of which can exacerbate your pain, fatigue, and other symptoms.

There are answers! The key to managing any stress is to recognize the signs and symptoms and minimize these before you become overwhelmed. You have read Steps 1 to 5 and, I hope, should be feeling more in control of your arthritis pain and other symptoms. In Step 6, I will explain how to identify your arthritis stressors and symptoms and give you ways to regain control of all aspects of life.

The Power of the Mind

Have you ever stepped on a piece of glass and not thought anything of it until you saw blood? Then suddenly your pulse quickened, and the wound throbbed in rhythm with your heartbeat. Doctors know that the mind can accentuate—or diminish—the pain you feel, depending on how

Gather Your Pain-Free Tools

1. In your Pain-Free Diary, schedule periodic time-outs throughout the day and week so you can practice the mind/body exercises in this step.
2. Record the exercises you like best and write down your responses after doing each relaxation technique. When the anxiety of painful flare-ups causes stress hormones to skyrocket, you can use mind/body therapies to relax before other stress symptoms occur.
3. Keep a list of CDs that you enjoy listening to and write down your emotional and pain response after a listening session.
4. Use the Pain-Free Diary to record your feelings about arthritis, your pain, and any limitations you have. Reread these thoughts weeks later and see if you are conquering any fears or frustrations as your Pain-Free Program results in less pain and increased mobility.

Signs and Symptoms of Stress

Stress symptoms vary greatly from one person to the next, but besides feeling pressured or overwhelmed, other symptoms include:
- Physical complaints—stomach aches, headaches, diarrhea
- Problems getting along with others
- Changes in behavior at home—temper outbursts, unexplained anger, crying for no reason
- Regression—behavior that is not age-appropriate
- Sleep patterns—nightmares, too little or too much sleep
- Communication difficulty—your personality takes a change; e.g., a withdrawn person suddenly requires much attention or an extrovert becomes withdrawn
- Impatience—you seem to have a short circuit in behavior
- Substance abuse—increased use of alcohol or drugs

you perceive it. In this step, I'll teach you how to use your mind—mental distraction—to de-stress your body and thus reduce your joint or muscle pain. If left untreated, chronic stress and anxiety may lead to depression, along with a host of other problems (see page 135). Nevertheless, there are some pain-free mind power strategies for resolving these feelings before they overwhelm you.

Check Your Attitude

Although arthritis is limiting, you can do a lot to keep it from controlling your entire life. In this regard, positive thinking goes a long way as you focus on wellness—not pain or illness. Through years of research, we know that optimists do better than pessimists in work, school, and sports. Optimists have lower rates of depression and stress-related illnesses, and actually live longer.

Recent studies in the field of psychoneuroimmunology (mind-body interplay) link pessimism and a negative attitude with decline of immune function and poor health. A revealing thirteen-year study at the National Center for Health Statistics found that those who were pessimistic were 1.5 times likelier to die of heart disease than optimists were, even when other risk factors were taken into account.

When you add to a pessimistic personality the traits of cynicism and hostility, you have the perfect breeding ground for illness. At the 1997 meeting of the American Psychological Association, researchers from Bowling Green State University reported that cynicism, like depression and anxiety, can cause stress hormones to flow into the bloodstream, which can damage the cells that make up your immune system.

Pessimism Increases Pain Levels

Over the past twenty-five years, I've seen that arthritis patients who are negative or pessimistic seem to have higher levels of pain and greater limitations than those who are positive—in spite of the severity of arthritis. One patient I'll call Ben never started an exercise program because, as he put it, he just knew it would not work and could even worsen his osteoarthritis in the hip. Ben limped for several years before he finally had hip surgery because of the pain, stiffness, and immobility. Nonetheless, this invasive procedure and lengthy rehabilitation could have been postponed or even avoided had Ben willingly started exercise when he was first diagnosed.

In a study published in June 2002 in the *Journal of Behavioral Medicine*, researchers confirmed this mood-pain link, reporting that pessimistic people claim to have more knee pain and worse functioning than those with similar knee problems without such a negative outlook. In a study from Wake Forest University in Winston-Salem, North Carolina, researchers found that a negative outlook affects the physical health of a person, particularly when the worst outcome is expected.

Researchers measured physical pain, functioning, and outlook in 480 arthritis patients, who were at least sixty-five years old. All of the patients had arthritis knee pain most of the time, which caused disability. In surveys, researchers measured physical functioning and disability from pain. They also watched the participants engage in daily activities. They measured mood or outlook by asking participants if they agreed or disagreed with statements such as "I always look on the bright side of things" or "If something can go wrong for me, it will."

Researchers concluded that arthritis patients who were pessimistic were less able than their optimistic counterparts were to do activities such as walking, lifting an object, and climbing stairs, among others. Although optimistic participants were no better able to perform most activities than the other patients, they did have a positive attitude and were at least willing to try to improve their condition. The researchers concluded that if pessimistic people do not believe things will work out for them, they never try to achieve anything. Because of this, pessimistic people may not try to exercise or keep up with their fitness conditioning and thus feel more pain and immobility than their more positive counterparts.

I've found that patients who are optimistic in spite of their pain have "hope" that a treatment will work and tackle new modalities with enthusiasm instead of dread. Contrary to this, more negative patients usually quit trying altogether because in their minds they have decided that treatments such as an exercise regimen, frequent moist heat applications, or combination medications simply will not work for them.

Is Laughter the Missing Link?

The results of a variety of studies now provide mounting evidence that laughter may be one of the missing links for optimal health because it speeds production of new immune cells and reduces the stress hormone cortisol. In a highly sophisticated study, researchers discovered that the blood chemistry of professional actors actually changes during a performance. In one experiment, actors alternated between two plays, one depressing and one happy. The first play, *It's Cold Wanderer, It's Cold*, set during the Russian Revolution, was a drab, depressing piece about an assassin on the eve of his execution being questioned by the widow of the man he had murdered. At the end of this thirty-minute play, the actors went to their dressing rooms. Then, after a brief intermission, they returned.

This time, they starred in a stage adaptation of an *I Love Lucy* episode, with the "widow" now playing Lucy and the "assassin" now playing Ricky.

The actors repeated this staging over a two-week period, during which time researchers took blood samples from the actors after each performance with astonishing results. They found that simply by acting depressed, the actors had depressed their immune systems. However, when they returned to acting happy, their blood chemistry returned to healthy levels.

No, you don't have to be a Robin Williams to be able to summon positive emotions at will. Nevertheless, you may want to practice smiling if you are typically a toxic or critical person. Study after study shows that negative emotions such as pessimism, anger, mistrust, cynicism, and depression throw the immune system into a state that makes it harder to resist disease. Scientists have also found that negative people have burdened their immune systems and are more prone to develop certain diseases and then recover more slowly than their positive counterparts.

Learn to De-Stress

The main strategy in dealing with stress is to identify and remove or reduce its source. Identification may be relatively easy, but elimination is a challenge, especially when the source is a chronic disease such as arthritis. Knowing you have little control over your main stressor (arthritis pain), it is important to find simple ways to remove all other daily stress.

Stress comes with a host of signs and symptoms. For example, an acute or prolonged tense state may cause an increase in heart rate and blood pressure, dry mouth, enlarged pupils, sweaty palms, and fast, shallow "chest" breathing. However, mind-body exercises in this step help to break this tension cycle and enable bodily functions to return to normal. Allowing yourself time throughout the day to meditate, breathe deeply, or listen to music, among other methods, will help you to ease muscle tension and pain, as well as stay more relaxed.

Some of my patients find that mind-body exercises work within minutes of doing them. For example, deep abdominal breathing actually alters your psychological state, making a stressful moment diminish in intensity. Think about how your respiration quickens when you are fearful. Then consider how taking a deep, slow breath brings an immediate calming effect. Likewise, music therapy can lessen your heart rate on the first experience, if you mindfully focus on the music, rhythm, and resulting inner peace. Exercise, as discussed in Step 1, is a great stress reliever, and if you walk outdoors, you can benefit from the beauty and serenity of nature.

Focus on Spiritual Self-Care

For years, doctors have witnessed that patients who are more spiritual are better able to deal with the pain and other limitations of their chronic illnesses. While the diagnosis of arthritis may cause you to feel a loss of control of your life, spiritual coping strategies can enhance self-empowerment, helping you to regain control and find meaning and purpose in illness. Spirituality does not have to be synonymous with mainstream religion—you can have a spiritual awareness of the world around you without adhering to the doctrine of organized religion. For the purposes of this book, spirituality is where you place your belief, your source of hope, and where you seek harmony in life.

Acknowledging our spiritual nature enables us to feel part of something larger than ourselves, including a sense of community. Moreover, findings show that spiritual people may be healthier and have a more positive outlook on life. In the 1970s, Harvard cardiologist Herbert Benson, M.D., was the first physician to scientifically document the physiological benefits of meditation through his studies with practitioners of Transcendental Meditation. Thanks to the early theories of Benson and other brilliant researchers, many studies are focused on the mechanisms by which the mind and emotions affect physical well-being. For instance, in findings given at the May 2002 American Geriatrics Society's annual meeting, researchers at Johns Hopkins reported on a study to assess the connection between spirituality, disease severity, and perceptions of well-being in patients with chronic disease. In this study, seventy-seven patients aged thirty or older who had had rheumatoid arthritis for at least two years were evaluated. The scientists defined spirituality as "the capacity of a person to stand outside of his/her immediate sense of time and place and to view life from a larger, more detached perspective." Researchers found that spirituality did not reduce the problems with arthritis or decrease pain, but those people who were more spiritual were happier and had a more positive outlook on life.

Similar findings published in the April 2001 issue of the *Journal of Pain* revealed that spirituality might be a type of psychological resource that allows patients with rheumatoid arthritis to adjust better to living with a chronic illness. In a study done at Duke University in Durham, North Carolina, thirty-five people with rheumatoid arthritis were asked to keep daily diaries of their moods, religious and/or spiritual experiences, levels of pain, and coping strategies. Researchers concluded that the patients who were able to control and decrease pain using positive spiritual coping strategies were less likely to experience joint pain and more likely to experience positive mood and higher levels of social support.

In another study on women with fibromyalgia, researchers from the University of Maryland study found that an eight-week program of mindfulness meditation—combined with qigong (see page 147) and pain management counseling—resulted in a tremendous improvement in pain threshold, degree of anxiety and depression, coping, and overall daily function.

Spirituality is experienced in many ways—through relaxation, deep breathing, visualization, music, meditation, prayer, or journaling, among other modalities. Try the following mind/body therapies and write down those that help you feel more relaxed and give you a more positive perspective on life. If you need help in learning these therapies, talk with a licensed mental health counselor. Once you get used to doing these practices, lean on them regularly to decrease stress and increase spiritual awareness. Over time, you will begin to see life and your chronic pain in a more positive way.

The Relaxation Response

In his studies, Benson found that there was a counterbalancing mechanism to the fight-or-flight response, the primal response that causes the heart rate to soar, causes blood pressure to rise, and puts us on red alert when life's stressors are overwhelming. Just as stimulating an area of the hypothalamus can cause the stress response, so activating other areas of the brain results in its reduction. This study led to the discovery of the "relaxation response," a physiological state of inner quiet and peacefulness, a calming of negative thoughts and worries, and a mental focus away from the pain itself. Once your mind reaches a state of deep calm and relaxation, the body can relax and muscle tension subsides. This results in less pain. There are many mind-body or spiritual techniques that elicit the relaxation response, which I will explain later on.

Relaxation is defined by decreased muscle tension and respiration, lower blood pressure and heart rate, and improved circulation. The relaxation response slows down the sympathetic nervous system leading to:

- Decreased heart rate
- Decreased blood pressure
- Decreased sweat production
- Decreased oxygen consumption

- Decreased catecholamine production (dopamine and norepinephrine or brain chemicals associated with the stress response)
- Decreased cortisol production (stress hormone)

Relaxation can offer a real potential to reduce physical strain and emotional, negative thoughts—and increase your ability to fall asleep in less time. It appears to affect the pain experience by releasing endorphins—the body's natural opiates or pain-relieving hormones that are related to synthetic opiates like morphine.

How can you learn the relaxation response? Try these easy steps:

1. Set aside a period of about 20 minutes that you can devote to relaxation practice.
2. Remove outside distractions that can disrupt your concentration: turn off the radio, the television, even the ringer on the telephone, if need be.
3. Lie flat on a bed or floor, or recline comfortably so that your whole body is supported, relieving as much tension or tightness in your muscles as you can. You can use a pillow or cushion under your head if this helps.
4. During the 20-minute period, remain as still as possible; try to focus your thoughts as much as possible on the immediate moment, and eliminate any outside thoughts that may compete for your attention.
5. As you go through these steps, in your own way try to imagine that every muscle in your body is now becoming loose, relaxed, and free of any excess tension. Picture all of the muscles in your body beginning to unwind; imagine them beginning to go loose and limp.
6. Concentrate on making your breathing even. As you exhale, picture your muscles becoming even more relaxed, as if you somehow breathe the tension away. At the end of 20 minutes, take a few moments to focus on the feelings and sensations you have achieved. Notice whether areas that felt tight and tense at first now feel more loose and relaxed, and whether any areas of tension or tightness remain.

Eliciting the relaxation response in conjunction with music therapy, deep abdominal breathing, or other mind-body modality described in this step is an added bonus in reducing the emotional stress of daily living and easing tension-related muscle pain.

Deep Abdominal Breathing

Think about how your respiration quickens when you are fearful or in great pain and how taking a deep, slow breath can be a calming effect, reducing both stress and levels of muscle pain. Breathing is one of the few activities of the body that we can consciously control, and it can measure and alter your psychological state, making a stressful moment accelerate or diminish in intensity. Deep breathing also helps to diminish the stress response by oxygenating the blood and lowering blood pressure, and it calms the analytical mind.

Lie comfortably on your back in a quiet room with no distractions. Place your hands on your abdomen, and take in a slow, deliberate deep breath through your nostrils. If your hands are rising and your abdomen is expanding, then you are breathing correctly. If your hands do not rise, yet your chest is rising, you are breathing incorrectly.

Inhale to a count of five, then pause for three seconds. Now exhale to a count of five. You can start with ten repetitions of this exercise, then increase to twenty-five, twice daily. Use deep breathing exercises any time you feel overwhelmed throughout your day.

Progressive Muscle Relaxation

Many of my patients benefit from progressive muscle relaxation, also known as deep muscle relaxation. This mind-body exercise involves concentrating on different muscle groups as you contract and then relax all of the major muscle groups in the body, those of the head, neck, arms, chest, back, stomach, pelvis, legs, and feet.

To do progressive muscle relaxation, focus on each set of muscles, tense these muscles to the count of ten, then release to the count of ten. Along with progressive muscle relaxation, you might find added benefit with deep abdominal breathing, breathing in while tensing the muscles, and breathing out while relaxing them. The more relaxed your muscles are, the less pain you are likely to feel.

The good news about progressive muscle relaxation is that you can do it while lying in bed at night. If you awaken frequently, teach your body how to relax itself using this tool. You may find that this tool helps to calm you down so that sleep happens easily.

Visualization

Are you a daydreamer? Daydreaming is an excellent way of removing yourself from the stressors at hand. Marianne, a forty-two-year-old patient with rheumatoid arthritis, found visualization (also called guided imagery) to be an easily learned form of daydreaming that can be done anywhere—at any time—to create a desired state of relaxation in your mind. This mother of three took time-outs periodically during her busy day to visualize a scenic mountain view. Not only did the imaginary "trips" to the mountains help to ease daily stress, but she felt this day-dreaming time eased painful flares when she felt them coming on. Use the following steps to practice visualization:

1. Find a place where you can be comfortable and undisturbed for 15 minutes. Take the phone off the hook, and close the door so you can have no disturbances. If you are at work, let a co-worker know that you do not wish to be disturbed. (I had one patient who said after seeing the difference it made in his outlook and productivity on the job, his coworkers started doing visualization in their cubicles!)

2. While sitting or lying down, close your eyes, and take several deep breaths, using the instructions on page 141. Imagine a relaxing place—somewhere you have been before, such as watching a majestic sunset at the beach, sitting next to a babbling mountain stream, or lazily floating on a raft as the river current pushes you downstream.

3. Continue to breathe slowly and keep this relaxing image in your mind. As you explore the imaginary picture of your relaxing place, visualize all the stress and muscle tension leaving your body. Feel your surroundings—the wind, sun, and temperature. See the colors surrounding you. What sounds do you hear? Smell the freshness of the air. Touch the gentleness of the moment. Take in all the sensory details of your relaxing place and continue to de-stress.

4. After about 15 minutes, slowly open your eyes and acclimatize yourself to the surroundings in the room. Stretch your arms and legs; gently move your head from side to side and feel the tension release. Carry the calm feeling you now have with you through the day.

5. If you have trouble imagining scenes and images, purchase post-cards with peaceful, serene scenes on them, and keep these in your

desk. Use these cards when you need to remove yourself from the tension of daily life and imagine being in your circle of quiet where life is less threatening.

Music Therapy

Music may be enjoyable but some new research suggests that it might help with pain control. According to a study presented in September 2002 by Austrian researchers at the Tenth World Congress on Pain, music may be used effectively to ease tense muscles and relax the body—resulting in a decrease in pain perception.

Researchers divided a group of sixty-five patients with chronic low back pain into two groups. Roughly half the participants listened to music for twenty-five minutes each day, using headphones. The others did not listen to music. After three weeks, the patients who listened to music, along with doing relaxation exercises, had substantively reduced pain and also fewer sleep problems related to pain. Researchers concluded that calming music and classical pieces seemed to work best to ease tension and stress.

You can use music therapy to boost relaxation or to decrease anxiety if your stress levels mount. Many patients enjoy using headphones with favorite songs playing during exercise to help ease boredom and ensure they finish their daily Exercise Treatment. Some patients tell of music helping to distract them during painful arthritis flares. It can also reduce muscle tension by masking disturbing thoughts.

When you're under stress, your body releases epinephrine, norepinephrine, and other compounds that set your heart racing. If you are highly stressed and have trouble relaxing at bedtime, certain types of music can help transport your brain into the alpha wave, the state of relaxation much like meditation. All you need to implement music therapy is a CD or tape player, favorite CDs, and tapes. In choosing music to de-stress, try to find arrangements that have one beat per second with many low tones and a lot of strings. Find music that matches your personal moods and tastes, and use it to increase relaxation and soothing sleep, or keep you entertained during exercise.

Meditation

The use of meditation as a spiritual tool to alleviate pain and promote healing goes back thousands of years. Focusing the mind continuously on one word or phrase for a short period of time leads the body into the relaxation response with reductions in heart rate, blood pressure, respiratory rate, and muscle tension. Researchers surmise that meditation brings the brain wave pattern into an alpha state, which is a level of consciousness that promotes the healing state. Alpha brain waves are non-arousal (that is, non-alert) and slower than beta brain waves, which are arousal (alert) and hyper-alert. (For instance, if you just finished taking a test and then walked outside to enjoy the sunset, you'd probably be in alpha state. If you were in a serious debate with someone, you'd probably be in beta state.)

To practice meditation, sit comfortably with eyes closed and mentally repeat a word or sound (mantra) for 15 to 20 minutes, twice a day. Meditation is a cleansing process that allows you to be *mindful of the moment* without reacting to what you observe, see, or hear. Mindfulness is a moment-to-moment nonjudgmental awareness. At the heart of Buddhist meditation, mindfulness is ultimately about paying attention and cultivating clarity of mind, compassion, and self-love.

With practice, you'll find that you can lengthen the time of meditation and enjoy the stress reduction and healing benefits. Proponents of meditation find that it helps to de-stress and gives them a clearer understanding of their surroundings.

Meditative techniques are a key element in the Arthritis Self-Help Course at Stanford University. More than 100,000 people with arthritis have taken the twelve-hour course and learned meditation-style relaxation exercises as part of a comprehensive self-care program. Graduates report a 15 to 20 percent reduction in pain.

Prayer
Prayer is another spiritual modality that is popular among many arthritis sufferers. Not only does prayer allow your thoughts to take a break from daily analytical routines, but it helps to strengthen the spiritual dimension of life. Like meditation, prayer evokes the relaxation response that helps to calm anxiety, quiet the body, and promote inner healing. Prayer involves repetition of sounds, words, and meaningful petitions. When you pray or meditate, your body switches from the emergency "fight or flight" reaction, as it prepares to escape from a dangerous situation or animal, into a calmer, more peaceful mood. Studies show that prayer produces alpha waves consistent with serenity and happiness and helps to provide nourishment for your soul.

In a study published in the December 2000 issue of the *Journal of Holistic Nursing,* researchers from the University of Florida and Wayne

State University found that most older adults use prayer more than any other alternative health remedy to help manage the stress in their lives. In addition, nurse researchers found that prayer is the most frequently reported alternative treatment used by seniors to feel better or maintain health in general. In the report, 96 percent of older adults use prayer to specifically cope with stress, and 84 percent of the respondents reported using prayer more than other alternative remedies to feel better or to maintain their health. From a list of thirty-two alternative therapies, prayer is used more often than exercise, heat, relaxation techniques, humor, or herbal remedies to maintain overall health.

Journaling

An interesting study published in April 1999 in the *Journal of the American Medical Association* found writing about feelings and emotions to be therapeutic for those with chronic illnesses. In the study, researchers asked patients with asthma and arthritis to write about the most stressful event in their lives for a set time. These patients were compared with asthma and arthritis patients who were told to write about their plans for the day. Researchers found that 47 percent of the patients who wrote about their feelings showed clinical improvements after four months, compared with 24 percent in the control group. Asthma patients' lung functioning improved by an average of 19 percent, while the control group showed no change. And arthritis patients noted an average 28 percent reduction in the severity of their symptoms, compared with no change in the control group. It was theorized that writing about emotions helped patients cope with stressful problems, which is indicative that the "mind really matters."

Use your Pain-Free Diary to write down feelings about arthritis and the limitations you experience. Keeping a journal is therapeutic, and there are no rules attached. You can elaborate on your innermost feelings and fears and the limitations you feel with a chronic illness.

Ancient Healing Disciplines

Along with spiritual mind-body therapies, I'm a strong believer in ancient healing disciplines that can give a spiritual awareness and help you to find meaning in life. Yoga, tai chi, and qigong are all known to reduce stress, decrease pain, and increase positive thinking, as well as keep you limber and flexible.

Yoga

Many of my patients are avid proponents of yoga, taking group classes at the local gym or at exercise facilities in the area. One osteoarthritis patient, Lucy, age sixty-eight, started taking yoga two years ago. Today she has no morning stiffness and is able to do almost anything she wants without limitations from painful joints or fatigue. "With yoga, I sleep better, I'm more flexible, and my mood has greatly improved," Lucy said.

Yoga, an ancient Indian practice, has survived the ages and is now popular in Western nations. It is estimated that more than 20 million Americans now practice yoga. For those with arthritis, the various slow motion postures and deep breathing exercises help to integrate the body, breath, and mind, and may help ease pain and stiffness, as well as alleviate emotional stress.

Several small studies on the use of yoga with osteoarthritis of the hands and carpal tunnel syndrome were published in the February 2000 issue of the journal *Rheumatic Diseases Clinics of North America*. In these studies, researchers found that yoga gives greater reduction in pain than in those who did not practice yoga. Yoga also helps to ease stress and to increase relaxation and an awareness of the body. For instance, in a study on yoga and chronic pain from Harbor-UCLA Medical Center in Torrance, California, researchers found that Iyengar yoga, a type of yoga that combines breathing exercises with difficult poses, may help older adults alleviate the chronic pain of arthritis.

Because yoga improves muscle strength and involves stretching and relaxation postures, it should provide healing advantages for those with rheumatoid arthritis and other inflammatory conditions, as well as for those with fibromyalgia. In a 1994 study published in the *British Journal of Rheumatology*, researchers found that twenty patients with rheumatoid arthritis had left-hand grip strength improve significantly after doing yoga postures. All volunteers in the study wanted to continue the yoga classes after the study was completed.

Some of yoga's pain-relieving and healing benefits:

>Boosts flexibility
>Increases range of motion in joints
>Strengthens the spine
>Firms abdominal muscles
>Removes body tension
>Improves posture

Reduces anxiety
Lowers blood pressure
Improves respiratory function
Boosts self-confidence

Yoga's physical postures (*asanas*) are helpful in moving your joints in range of motion. The slow, gentle stretches help to lubricate the joints and send nutrients and oxygen to the muscles, bathing them in fresh blood. Taking time to relax and enjoy stretching helps to reduce your blood pressure and relieves stress. Just make sure the type of yoga you choose is not taxing. Ashtanga yoga, an extreme style of yoga, is a demanding series of asansas that will leave you breathless and possibly aching.

Two yoga exercises that I find particularly helpful for those with arthritis include the Flower (see figure 6.1), a great exercise for those with arthritis of the hands, and the Corpse (figure 6.2), which helps to stretch the entire body, easing minor aches and pains.

Call your local support group or gym, and ask about a special yoga class for those with arthritis. Instructional videos are also available that can help you learn the basic beginner postures in the privacy of your own home.

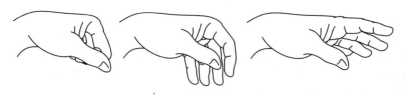

Figure 6.1.

The Flower

Make a tight fist and hold for six seconds. Then slowly release the grip and open your hand, stretching your figures as you count off six seconds. Do this with both hands, several times daily, or when your fingers feel tight and achy.

Qigong

Tagged as the "mother of Chinese self-healing," qigong (pronounced chee-gong) is said to be one of the most powerful healing traditions ever developed in human history. Qi means air, breath, or vital essence; gong means work, self-discipline, achievement, or mastery. This healing

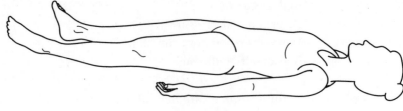

Figure 6.2.

The Corpse

Lie on your back on a comfortable surface, and stretch your arms and legs out straight. Keep your arms down by your sides, and extend your legs straight from the hips. Your feet should be about twelve inches apart, with both feet turned out slightly to keep the feet, ankles, and legs relaxed. With palms facing upward, keep the arms eight to ten inches from the body. Lengthen the back on the floor and feel all muscles stretching and releasing. Notice your shoulder blades and hips, and adjust the body until you feel balanced on both the left and right sides of the body. Scan your body and consciously relax every muscle group, including the throat, face, and eye muscles. Continue this scanning as you lie down and relax, and become aware of areas in which you might hold chronic tension. As you lie there, feel your breathing take you into a deeper relaxed state.

tradition combines aerobic conditioning, isometrics, isotonics, meditation, and relaxation techniques. Because it involves specific physical postures that dissolve tension, the practice of qigong triggers a wide array of physiological mechanisms, which have profound healing benefits:

- Delivers oxygen to the tissues
- Eliminates waste products and aids in transporting immune cells through the lymph system
- Shifts the chemistry of the brain and the nervous system

There are at least a thousand varieties of qigong, yet all focus on getting *qi*, or energy, moving smoothly through the body. When *qi* is obstructed, you will have fatigue and illness.

Proponents of qigong claim that this discipline increases energy, decreases fatigue, and alleviates pain. Some believe that it can help to heal back pain, carpal tunnel syndrome, circulatory problems, depression, high blood pressure, insomnia, symptoms of menopause, neuralgia, chronic pain, and TMJ (tempero mandibala joint) syndrome.

Experts conclude that *qi* has to be cultivated daily, so the rudimentary exercises should be done each morning to build *qi*. You may have to pay a practitioner to teach you qigong, but once you understand the postures and breathing regimen, you can do it at any time at no cost. Some people feel results instantaneously, while for others it may take days or weeks before a difference is noticed in mood, energy, and wellness.

Tai Chi

Tai chi is a centuries-old Chinese martial art that was used for defense. Today, millions around the world practice tai chi for its meditative and strengthening benefits. This ancient discipline consists of a series of set motions that require you to move your arms, legs, and torso slowly and gracefully. Because you learn to stand and balance on one foot in tai chi, this popular exercise aids in increasing equilibrium and flexibility, helping to prevent falls.

A study from Emory University published in 1996 in the *Journal of the American Medical Association* evaluated various types of exercise and reported that tai chi produced significant decreases in the risk of falling when compared to other activities. In another study, published in 2001 in the *Annals of Behavioral Medicine*, researchers concluded that older adults can lower their blood pressure and ease arthritis symptoms through tai chi. Other findings presented at the annual meeting of the American College of Rheumatology in December 2001 by researchers from South Korea reported similar results. These scientists found that tai chi may help some with arthritis, making it easier to move and get through daily activities. At the end of the two-week study, women in the tai chi group reported less pain, fewer difficulties with daily activities, improved balance, and greater abdominal muscle strength.

To find an experienced tai chi instructor in your area, call your local support group or gym.

Biofeedback

If after trying some of the mind-body or spiritual tools in this chapter you are still having a lot of muscle tension, increased pain, or trouble calming down or sleeping because of daily stress, you may want to look into biofeedback. Biofeedback can allow you to have conscious control over body functions that usually occur automatically—the heartbeat, blood pressure, muscle tension, pain response, and brain waves.

With biofeedback, you are connected to a machine that informs you and a professional therapist when you are physically tensing and relaxing your body. You will learn through "feedback" how to control your heart rate, blood pressure, and muscle tension. Tension in the muscles and joints is a normal reaction to arthritis pain, but too much tension can actually increase your sensitivity to the pain. With sensors placed over specific muscle sites, the therapist will read the tension in your muscles, heart rate, breathing pattern, the amount of sweat produced, or body temperature. Any one or all these readings can let the therapist know if you are learning to relax.

Studies have shown that people who received biofeedback treatments had fewer tender points, and lower pain intensity and morning stiffness. Eventually people who have had biofeedback can recognize their own physical reactions to stress without the feedback, and can modify their behavior accordingly.

Counseling

The role of psychological counseling in your Pain-Free Program is to help you develop appropriate and workable coping strategies to deal with your arthritis and the limitations you face. Psychological intervention is an accepted component for everyone—not just those who have "psychological problems." Most of my patients find that counseling often provides excellent coping methods that can be used daily. Many patients find that counseling often serves as the social support that is so necessary to stay strong during times of crisis or illness. For instance, family and friends frequently offer unsolicited advice ("Are you sure you're really in pain . . .?") and frequently fail to recognize the severity of the impact of arthritis. A therapist trained in pain management understands what you are going through and can give you strategies to help you live positively. Some therapists offer couples groups to help with marital adjustments; others offer support groups to relieve the sense of isolation, or psychoeducational groups (e.g., stress management, relaxation) to teach coping skills.

You might find one of these options helpful:

• Individual counseling—a one-on-one session with a therapist in which individual problems are addressed.

- Family counseling—a session with the therapist, you, and your family so others can be involved in understanding your limitations and the impact these may have on your family's lifestyle.
- Group counseling—a group session with others who live with arthritis or chronic pain where you can share feelings as well as coping strategies.

I've found that patients who lack social support suffer tremendously from loneliness, fear, and disconnection. That's why reaching out and seeking support from experts as well as those who live with arthritis is

Check Signals for Depression

Living with chronic pain can cause depression with feelings of hopelessness, uncontrollable tearfulness, and loss of self-worth. While many individuals may have one or more of these symptoms at one time or another, it becomes a problem when depression symptoms continue on a daily basis for at least two weeks.

Check out the following common signals for depression. If you have any of these signals, talk with your doctor about treatment. Often depression is temporary, especially with a chronic illness such as arthritis. If needed, there are many excellent prescription drugs and many medical protocols that can help greatly.

Common Signals for Depression
- Disturbances in sleep patterns
- Loss of interest in usual activities
- Weight loss or gain (more than 5 percent of body weight)
- Fatigue
- Impaired thinking
- Thoughts of dying or suicide
- Depressed thoughts or irritability
- Mood swings
- Staying at home all the time
- Avoidance of special friends
- Difficulty concentrating
- Difficulty getting out of bed
- Feelings of worthlessness or excessive or inappropriate guilt
- Agitation or, in contrast, a general slowing of intentional bodily activity

Let's Review: 8 Steps for Getting Started with Mind-Body Exercises

1. Talk to your doctor about your stress level. If your anxiety is high or if you feel depressed, ask if medications may be necessary or might help ease symptoms.

2. A common mistake made by many when they use alternative therapies is that they stop traditional medical treatment altogether. If your doctor has prescribed medication for depression, anxiety, insomnia, or other stress-related condition, continue this treatment while learning alternate methods of stress reduction.

3. Visualize yourself as free of pain. Although this is not easy—it takes a commitment to "positive thinking"—it can help you feel better— fast.

4. Stay the course. Even if you think the mind-body or spiritual tools are not working for you, continue to stay focused on stress reduction and incorporate the practices in your daily routine.

5. Avoid diversions during your stress-reduction time. Let family and friends know that you need time alone to do your mind/body exercises. (They will appreciate your positive mood after you've spent time relaxing!)

6. Realize that we live in an imperfect world, so eliminate the word perfect from your vocabulary. Give yourself permission to be good enough. This will help you accept your humanness and reduce the unnecessary stress you put on yourself to be all things to all people.

7. If you are a negative thinker, filled with worries and fears, make an appointment with a licensed mental health counselor. Talking to a professional can help you analyze and counter negative thoughts that make you depressed. Negativity can keep you from moving forward with your life.

8. For a double benefit in pain relief and stress reduction, continue to use the Exercise Treatment as outlined in this program.

an important part of moving to pain-free living. Although you cannot control your diagnosis, you can create a strong network of doctors, family, and friends who will be there for you—on good days and bad. Studies confirm that people with strong social supports tend to fare better in every life situation, particularly when confronted with a serious illness.

Doctor's Pain-Free Treatment

Using the mind-body or spiritual therapies described in this step, select those exercises that you will enjoy and practice them. As you become proficient with these mental aerobics and incorporate them in your daily life, your body will automatically switch from the pumping "fight or flight" response of high stress into a calmer, more peaceful mood.

Remember, the stress of a chronic illness such as arthritis can undermine any control you might have had. Use the methods in this step to restore calm and composure and become the master of your pain.

Osteoarthritis
- Practicing the relaxation response or another method to achieve relaxation (deep breathing, progressive muscle relaxation, meditation) can help pain control. Be sure to allow time daily to do these mind-body exercises.
- Tai chi or yoga (with adjustments if your joint movements are limited by arthritis) is great for stability, improvement in flexibility, and pain control.

Fibromyalgia
- Because of the stress associated with FMS, it is important to find the mind-body techniques that work with your busy lifestyle. Try each of the techniques listed and rate them in your Pain-Free Diary. Then, focus on the exercises that bring you the best results in decreasing anxiety, increasing restful sleep, and alleviating muscle pain.
- Yoga, qigong, or tai chi may help increase your flexibility, stretch muscles, and ease unending stress.
- Because depression is so common with FMS, consider counseling so this problem will not limit your improvement.

Carpal Tunnel Syndrome
- Use the Flower yoga posture (see page 147) frequently throughout your day to ease muscle tension in the hand and wrist.

Bursitis/Tendonitis
- To improve your flexibility and strength, find a yoga, qigong, or tai chi class in your area. Practicing these ancient disciplines can help ease pain and also prevent future injuries or pain.

Rheumatoid Arthritis (and Other Inflammatory Arthritis)

- Pain control can improve tremendously with relaxation response practice. Review the discussed mind-body tools and find the one that works best for you.
- Start a journal in which you describe the emotions you have about your arthritis. Write about your fears and frustrations, the limitations you experience, and questions you might have about the future of living with a chronic illness. See if journaling helps to alleviate unnecessary stress and frees you to move forward in your pain-free goals.
- Yoga, qigong, and tai chi all improve flexibility, strength, and steadiness. Call your local support group to see if special classes are available for those with rheumatoid arthritis.
- If your chronic pain has led to depression, talk to a licensed mental health counselor. Seeking help early on in the disease can help you to avoid problems associated with depression and other mood disorders.

Choose the Latest Medical Treatments

We have certainly come a long way in our diagnosis and treatment of arthritis over the last hundred years, and the majority of medical break-throughs have been in the last decade. Of course, most people with arthritis know that medications can be a necessary component for ending pain and stiffness. Even if you haven't taken prescription arthritis medications, you've probably looked for relief with one of the over-the-counter pain relievers.

In Steps 1 to 6, you learned why exercise, diet, lifestyle changes, alternative therapies, massage, and mind-body tools are instrumental in keeping pain and inflammation at bay. The last step of the Pain-Free Program will help you learn how to use the right medications for your particular type of arthritis, so you can live an active life again.

All Arthritis Medications Are Not the Same

I'll never forget when forty-one-year-old Caroline was diagnosed with rheumatoid arthritis and her first response was that she'd take over-the-counter ibuprofen, a nonsteroidal anti-inflammatory drug (NSAID). "My mother and sister live on ibuprofen for their osteoarthritis, and, after all, arthritis medication is arthritis medication."

Maybe, maybe not. I explained to my patient that while some medications such as the NSAIDs can help ease symptoms of many types of arthritis, other excellent pharmaceuticals are specifically designed to treat just one type of arthritis. For example, because of the destructive nature of rheumatoid arthritis, this inflammatory type of arthritis requires a more specific medication that can actually stop or delay the progress and destruction. Some medications, such as the biologic medications, may achieve this goal. In addition, gout, another common form of inflammatory arthritis, may respond quickly to an NSAID or colchicine. Attacks can also be prevented with allopurinol, another commonly used medication for gout.

Your Medication Resource

No matter which type of arthritis you have, you'll find Step 7 to be an excellent pharmaceutical resource to increase your awareness of treatment options. To help you understand the types of treatment, I will begin with information on the basic analgesics and anti-inflammatory drugs, which can help relieve mild to moderate arthritis pain. Then I'll give detailed information on the latest medications for the more serious forms of this disease, such as rheumatoid arthritis. At the end of Step 7, I'll outline the most commonly used medications with the Doctor's Pain-Free Treatment.

Use the information in this step as a tool to ensure you get the best possible medication for your arthritis pain and other symptoms. Talk to your doctor about which drug may give you the most benefit with fewest side effects. Knowledge about possible treatment options can give you more control over your illness. In doing so, you will start on the path to optimal health and a more pain-free, active life.

Gather Your Pain-Free Tools

1. In your Pain-Free Diary, record all the medications you take. Write down any side effects you feel, including symptoms such as fatigue, nausea, stomach pain, indigestion, light-headedness, or insomnia.
2. Write down medications you've taken in the past for arthritis and any effect or side effect you experienced.
3. Take the Pain-Free Diary with you to your next doctor's visit. Talk about the medications and side effects. Ask your doctor if one of the new medications might help your type of arthritis. If you try different medications, be sure to keep a written log of each one, along with how you felt before, during, and after taking it.

Med Alert

Always follow the directions on the medication label, unless your doctor directs otherwise. If you are taking another medication prescribed by a different doctor, check with your pain doctor first to make sure you won't have a drug-drug interaction.

Commonly Used Over-the-Counter Analgesics

Brand Name	Generic Name
Advil	ibuprofen
Anadin	aspirin (with caffeine)
Bayer and other brands	aspirin
Motrin	ibuprofen
Mycoprin	enteric-coated asprin
Neurofen	ibuprofen
Nu-Seal	enteric-coated asprin
Panadol	paracetamol

Mild to Moderate Pain

Over-the-Counter Aspirin, Paracetamol, Ibuprofen, Naproxen

WHAT THEY'RE PRESCRIBED FOR

Over-the-counter analgesics, including aspirin, paracetamol, and low-dose ibuprofen or naproxen, are extremely effective in treating mild to moderate arthritis pain and stiffness. In fact, aspirin was used to treat pain as early as the fifth century B.C., when Hippocrates prescribed a bitter powder from the bark of a willow tree to treat aches and pains.

Aspirin and ibuprofen work by blocking the production of prostaglandins, those chemicals in the body that cause pain, inflammation, and swelling. Low doses of aspirin may ease the pain, but usually will not effectively stop the inflammation. Higher doses may be needed to reduce inflammation, and these doses can have serious side effects.

Paracetamol (Panadol) elevates the pain threshold, so you perceive less pain. Although paracetamol is often recommended for osteoarthritis, many doctors also prescribe this drug for pain that does *not* stem from inflammation, since it does not affect prostaglandins. Paracetamol can give temporary relief in arthritis pain, but usually the pain and swelling will eventually require other medicines. Of course, paracetamol can still be used as a supplemental medication for pain.

Over-the-Counter Ibuprofen

WHAT IT'S PRESCRIBED FOR

Ibuprofen is available over the counter for mild to moderate pain as a low dose of prescription-strength nonsteroidal anti-inflammatory drugs. When used as directed on the bottle label, side effects are usually low and the serious side effects (like peptic ulcer disease and bleeding) caused by high doses are uncommon. However, sometimes these low doses may not provide enough relief from pain and inflammation. In these cases, the prescription strength of this and similar NSAID medications are used—and the chance of side effects increases.

I have many osteoarthritis patients who find good pain relief with simple over-the-counter analgesics, especially if they follow the moist heat therapy and Exercise Treatment, outlined in Step 1, and use the other steps in the Pain-Free Program. Even if osteoarthritis only affects a few joints, the pain and stiffness can severely limit daily activities and the ability to exercise. However, when one of the recommended over-the-counter analgesics is added to the daily Pain-Free Program, the arthritis pain may no longer limit your activities—and more important, won't stop regular exercise.

POTENTIAL SIDE EFFECTS

In some people, aspirin can lead to heartburn, nausea, or vomiting, and increased clotting time for blood with easier bruising. If low doses are used, peptic ulcers with gastrointestinal bleeding are not common. Paracetamol is relatively free of side effects if taken according to package directions, but can cause liver and kidney damage, especially if taken in high doses. Ibuprofen can cause upset stomach, abdominal pain, peptic ulcers, anemia, and kidney disorders. If taken as directed on the bottle, side effects are uncommon with these lower doses.

POSSIBLE INTERACTIONS

Avoid taking paracetamol if you have more than three alcoholic drinks daily, as this combination may increase the potential for liver damage. Don't combine more than one NSAID medication unless your doctor

Commonly Used Traditional Nonsteroidal
Anti-inflammatory Drugs (NSAIDs)

Brand Name	Generic Name
Advil	ibuprofen
Arthrosin	naproxen
Arthrotec	diclofenac (plus Misoprostol)
Aspirin (many brand names)	aspirin products
Clinoril	sulindac
Fenopron	fenoprofen
Indocid	indomethacin
Naprosyn EC	naproxen (enteric-coated)
Naprosyn	naproxen
Nycopren	naproxen
Neurofen	ibuprofen
Oruvail	ketoprofen delayed release
Ponstan	metanamic acid
Preservex	aceclofenac
Relifex	nabumetone
Surgam	tenoxicam
Trilisate	choline magnesium trisalicylate
Voltarol	diclofenac

instructs you to do so. (If you take low-dose aspirin to help reduce the risk of heart attack and stroke, this may be added to your NSAID medication. But, check with your doctor to be sure it's right for you.)

Traditional Nonsteroidal Anti-inflammatory Drugs (NSAIDs)

WHAT THEY'RE PRESCRIBED FOR
Although one of the over-the-counter analgesic medications might give pain relief for a while, many people with osteoarthritis eventually find they need greater relief and turn to one of the nonsteroidal anti-inflammatory drugs by prescription.

All of the NSAID medications control pain and swelling in arthritis by blocking the body's production of prostaglandins—the chemicals that create inflammation, pain, swelling, and, in some cases, joint destruction. These medications work by blocking the action of cyclooxygenase (COX, the enzyme that produces prostaglandins), resulting in reduced pain and inflammation.

Aspirin and other traditional NSAIDs block prostaglandin production, slowing the unwanted effects of inflammation and reducing pain and stiffness. However, prostaglandins also send some good messages, protecting the stomach lining, controlling platelets (the cells that help blood clot), and helping kidney function. By blocking the actions of prostaglandins, aspirin and traditional NSAIDs also increase the risk of peptic ulcers, bleeding, and kidney damage. For those who take one of the traditional NSAIDs on a regular basis, there is a 2 to 4 percent chance of peptic ulcers and bleeding. Because these medications are so widely used, this creates a large number of peptic ulcers, hospitalizations, risks, and increased health expense. Some patients who take these drugs may also have an affect of reduced kidney function.

There are more than twenty-five NSAIDs available, and most people can find one that gives relief of pain without side effects. When I explain to patients that it might require trial and error to find the right medication, I always think of my patient Alice. This sixty-four-year-old woman tried seven different NSAIDs before finding one that relieved her pain completely and had few side effects. She'd try a new NSAID every two weeks, hoping it would be the one that worked. For weeks, the frustrated Alice had no luck, going through bottle after bottle of pills. Nevertheless, when she found the right medication, it began to give her relief within hours and continued to work as long as she stayed on that NSAID.

Because each person's response to medication differs, you will probably have to try several different NSAIDs before you find the one that gives you relief from pain and stiffness. While all of the NSAIDs have a similar average success rate in pain relief, you will need to find one with the best response for you.

To avoid getting a large supply of medications that may not work for your pain, ask your doctor for samples. Or, ask for a small, two-week prescription of the NSAID. If you take the NSAID for about fourteen days and there is no improvement in symptoms, or if you feel side effects, try a different one. Continue the medication that gives the most pain relief with the fewest side effects. In some cases, the pharmacist can even compound some NSAIDs into topical creams, gels, and ointments that are applied directly to the inflamed joint or muscle, which can reduce systemic side effects. Talk to your doctor if this seems like a more viable option for your pain.

POTENTIAL SIDE EFFECTS

Traditional NSAIDs are usually well tolerated, but you might experience indigestion, heartburn, peptic ulcer disease, abdominal pain, or intestinal bleeding. These side effects are more common in those who are over age sixty-five. In addition, those who are taking prednisone or have already had peptic ulcers or illnesses such as heart failure are at a higher risk for gastrointestinal problems with NSAIDs. Some new studies find that about 2 to 4 percent of people who take one of the traditional NSAIDs may develop complications of peptic ulcers such as intestinal bleeding. The bleeding most often comes without warning signs, requires hospitalization, and increases the risk of death.

Traditional NSAIDs should be used with caution if you have kidney or liver disease, congestive heart failure, high blood pressure, diabetes mellitus, SLE (systemic lupus erythematosus), asthma, or peptic ulcers. These should not be taken if you are taking anticoagulants, such as warfarin (Coumarin), or if you are pregnant.

Med Alert

The doses of aspirin, or ibuprofen sold over the counter and taken as directed usually do not cause stomach or intestinal bleeding. However, if you have had a peptic ulcer, if you're over age sixty-five, if you take prednisone, or if you have congestive heart failure, then higher doses of the medications listed in the table on page 159, might increase your risk of stomach complications and bleeding. As with any medication, check with your doctor before you take one of these.

If you must take a traditional NSAID, there are still ways to protect your stomach and avoid peptic ulcers, complications, and hospitalizations. Medications such as Losec (omeprazole), Zoton (lansoprazole), Aciphex (rabeprazole), Protonix (pantoprazole), Nexium (esomeprazole), and Misoporostol (cytotec) work to decrease acid production in the stomach and protect the stomach lining from the negative effects of the traditional NSAIDs. This extra medication (taken because of the first medication) can add expense to your treatment. Still, the benefit of preventing bleeding complications and hospitalization is worth the cost. If you find relief with one of the COX-2 NSAIDs listed on page 166, it is not necessary to routinely add one of the stomach protective medications.

If you take one of the NSAIDs regularly, your doctor will check blood tests for anemia, kidney, liver, and other studies for safety every few months.

If you have aspirin sensitivity, use NSAIDs with caution, as the medications are similar enough to cause reactions. For example, some people cannot take aspirin or NSAIDs because of the aspirin sensitivity that occurs in about 10 to 15 percent of people with asthma and 30 to 40 percent of those who have asthma and nasal polyps. You might feel such symptoms as itching, rashes, hives, swelling, nasal congestion, and wheezing. Talk to your doctor about alternative therapies for resolving pain if you have this sensitivity.

POSSIBLE INTERACTIONS
If one of these medications gives relief of pain and stiffness, it's usually safe if taken as directed. However, be sure that you don't have a hidden or unusual risk. For example, if you take warfarin (Coumarin) or other blood thinners, then aspirin or the nonsteroidal anti-inflammatories naproxen and ibuprofen should not be taken because of an increased risk of bleeding. Paracetamol is safe to use with warfarin. One of the COX-2 NSAIDs on page 166 can be combined with this blood thinner.

Don't combine more than one type of NSAID unless your doctor advises it. Alcohol increases the risk of peptic ulcers when combined with an NSAID. Especially if you're on multiple medications, your doctor should check your list to be sure an NSAID is a safe combination.

COX-2 NSAIDs
The new types of NSAIDs called COX-2 inhibitors mainly target the key COX enzyme to block inflammation and pain. Unlike the traditional NSAIDs, which can lead to serious gastrointestinal problems, including bleeding ulcers, the new COX-2 inhibitors have fewer side effects, especially peptic ulcers and bleeding. These COX-2 NSAIDs are used to treat osteoarthritis, fibromyalgia, bursitis and tendonitis, and rheumatoid and other inflammatory arthritis, among others. They are also used for other types of pain unrelated to arthritis, such as menstrual pain and pain after surgery or dental work.

To understand how COX-2 inhibitors or "super aspirins" work to reduce inflammation, let's take a step back in time. In the early 1970s researchers found that aspirin works by blocking the body's production of prostaglandins—the chemicals that cause inflammation, pain, and

Common Side Effects of NSAIDs

Abdominal pain
Abnormal liver tests (blood tests)
Asthma in those allergic to the drug
Bruising or bleeding more easily
Aggravation or cause of kidney (renal) failure
Diminished effect of diuretics
Dizziness
Gastritis
Heartburn
Increased blood pressure (hypertension)
Indigestion
Intestinal bleeding
Lower hemoglobin (anemia)
May affect other medications taken
May decrease platelet effect (can affect bleeding)
May change the effect of other medication, such as oral diabetic medications, warfarin (Coumarin), beta-blockers, ACE inhibitors, diuretics
Peptic ulcer
Ringing in the ears (tinnitus)
Sodium retention and edema in the feet and legs

swelling, and even joint destruction in some types of arthritis. In 1971, scientist John Vane showed in Nobel Prize-winning studies that aspirin inhibits the functioning of cyclooxygenase, or COX, an enzyme that cells need to make prostaglandins.

Prostaglandins send messages to trigger inflammation resulting in pain and swelling in arthritis. When traditional NSAIDs block all the prostaglandin actions, you have less pain and stiffness. Nonetheless, the good effects of prostaglandins are also blocked, including the necessary stomach protection. Therefore, while aspirin and traditional NSAIDs may give pain relief, they also leave you vulnerable to the risk of peptic ulcers and bleeding.

In the early 1990s scientists discovered that there were actually two forms of the COX enzyme cells needed to produce prostaglandins. The COX-1 enzyme was common in normal tissues and helped maintain the normal workings of tissues in the stomach, platelets, and kidneys, and the COX-2 form controlled inflammation and pain in joints and other

Less Common Side Effects of NSAIDs

Confusion
Constipation
Depression
Diarrhea
Difficulty sleeping
Fatigue
Headaches
Impaired thinking (uncommon, but occurs at times in older patients)
Itching
Lowered white cells in blood count
Meningitis-like illness (rare)
Mouth ulcers
Occasional blurred vision
Other individual allergic or unusual reactions
Palpitations
Rash
Sun sensitivity

areas. In this breakthrough discovery, scientists realized that the real target to stop inflammation and pain is the COX-2 enzyme.

All of the traditional NSAIDs on the market such as aspirin, ibuprofen, naproxen and the list of NSAIDs on page 159 target both COX-2 and COX-1. While blocking pain, these medications leave many vulnerable to serious side effects involving the stomach and kidneys.

The newer NSAIDs (COX-2 inhibitors, or super aspirin) only target the COX-2 enzyme. These medications give relief of inflammation and pain but still allow protection of the stomach lining, platelets, and kidneys. The COX-2 NSAIDs give the same chance of improvement in arthritis pain and swelling but with dramatically decreased risk of peptic ulcer and bleeding. COX-2 NSAIDs do not affect platelets, so other bleeding problems can also be avoided. In addition, it is usually not necessary to add one of the stomach-protective drugs when you take a COX-2 NSAID.

POTENTIAL SIDE EFFECTS
If you are allergic to sulfa antibiotics, avoid Celebrex or Bextra. There are occasional reports of abdominal pain, diarrhea, headache, indigestion, or

Treating Back Pain

More than half of all Americans suffer from back pain every year. Sometimes the pain hits suddenly without any particular incident to trigger it. Other times the pain is the result of an old injury or degenerative disease. These attacks may come two or three times a year. Back pain can cause many lost hours from work and daily activities. With treatment, about 80 to 90 percent of back pain cases improve after seven to ten days.

The exact causes of these attacks of back pain are not known, but perhaps the most common source is a combination of pain from the muscles, tendons, and other soft tissues in the back, along with osteoarthritis in the lumbar spine. Although not as common, sometimes a ruptured disc between the vertebrae in the spine can cause pressure on a nerve coming from the spine, which makes pain travel down one or both legs, called "true sciatica."

These severe back pain attacks are treated with moist heat (see page 14), such as a warm shower twice daily for 10 to 15 minutes, activity as limited by the pain, a gradual increase in back exercises, addition of one of the NSAIDs listed on page 159, and a pain medication, if needed for relief. It's almost never necessary to stay in bed for days; in fact, complete bed rest might delay your improvement. If necessary, a local injection of cortisone may speed up your improvement, if a painful trigger area remains. If the pain worsens each day or if you still have no relief after a week, talk with your doctor for further plans to find the exact cause of the pain.

nausea with the COX-2 NSAIDs. If you are taking an anticoagulant medication such as Coumarin (warfarin), use COX-2 inhibitors with caution. Although the risk of gastrointestinal bleeding is greatly reduced with COX-2 inhibitors, it is not totally eliminated. Check with your doctor if you have unexplained nausea or abdominal pain.

Otherwise, the most common side effects of the COX-2 NSAIDs are similar to those listed for the NSAIDs (see page 163). As with all NSAIDs, your doctor will check your blood pressure, monitor for edema (swelling from fluid) in the feet and legs, and order blood tests to check kidney function. Periodically, your doctor will evaluate other tests, including tests for anemia, tests of the liver, and routine tests for small amounts of blood in the stool that might not be detectable otherwise.

Commonly Used COX-2 NSAIDs

Brand Name	Generic Name
Arcoxia	etoricoxib
Celebrex	celecoxib
Bextra	valdecoxib
Mobic	meloxicam
Lodine	eledolac
Vioxx	rofecoxib

Aspirin and Your Heart

It is usually safe to combine a low dose of aspirin (81–325 mg daily) for its heart-protection effects when you take an NSAID. Keep in mind that even a low dose of aspirin slightly raises your chance of peptic ulcer and bleeding. Combined with an NSAID, this risk increases slightly but gives the benefit of reducing the risk of heart attack and stroke. Check with your doctor when you combine these drugs to be sure it's safe for you.

Some studies have suggested that patients who take COX-2 NSAIDs might have a higher risk of myocardial infarction (heart attack). So far, this is not proven, and tests are under way to find whether there is, in fact, any higher risk with these medications.

POSSIBLE INTERACTIONS
If you are taking an ACE inhibitor for hypertension, NSAIDs might increase your blood pressure slightly. If you are taking diflucan (Frusomide), lasix, lithium, or thiazide diuretics, talk to your doctor to see if this medication can be continued safely.

Corticosteroids (Cortisone Derivatives)

WHAT THEY'RE PRESCRIBED FOR
The cortisone medications are the strongest of the anti-inflammatory drugs. These medications block the production of prostaglandins and leukotrienes, as well as certain cytokines such as interleukin 1. Corticosteroids may be used daily; every other day; in short, high-dose "bursts"; or in tapered dosing. While they quickly reduce pain and

swelling, corticosteroids also have serious and unwanted side effects, if continued over a long period.

POSSIBLE SIDE EFFECTS

If you find it necessary to take prednisone, a corticosteroid, on a regular basis to control your arthritis, it's important to be aware of the potential side effects listed below. Using medication, your doctor can help you to control some of these effects, such as the increased risk of osteoporosis (bone thinning that can lead to fractures). For example, Fosamax (alendronate) or Actonel (risedronate) taken once weekly have been shown to prevent bone loss caused by prednisone. One of these medications is added for prevention if you must take prednisone in doses of 5–7.5 mg daily or higher for three months or longer.

The potential side effects with corticosteroids include the following:

> Weight gain
> Diarrhea or constipation
> Headache
> Increased or decreased appetite
> Increased sweating
> Nervousness
> Osteoporosis (bone thinning)
> Restlessness
> Difficulty sleeping
> Upset stomach
> Unusual or increased hair on the face/body
> Adrenal suppression
> Fluid and electrolyte disturbances
> Risk of gastritis
> Increased risk of infection
> Increase in blood glucose, especially in diabetes mellitus
> Emotional instability or psychosis

Joint injections of cortisone medications are safer. Because of their possible side effects, the cortisone medications are safer in arthritis treatment when given by occasional injection directly into the joint. The injected steroid medication gives quick relief, which begins within a few days and may last up to a few months. If you find relief with the injections, your doctor can safely repeat this treatment about every three months. Several different cortisone medications are available for injection and all are effective.

Consider cortisone injections if your arthritis is well controlled except for one or two joints. More than one joint can easily be injected at the same visit, if necessary. Your doctor can treat most joints with a cortisone medication, if necessary, for temporary relief of the pain.

Continue your basic program of moist heat, exercises, and other medications to control pain and stiffness. The injection targets just that particular joint, so the Pain-Free Program is important to keep pain down in other affected joints. Ask your doctor when you should resume exercises for the injected joint and when you can resume moist heat applications.

POSSIBLE INTERACTIONS

Corticosteroids are important medications that can affect the action of many other medications. The best advice is to make sure your doctor knows all of the medications you're taking, especially when a corticosteroid is added.

Commonly Used Corticosteroids

Brand Name	Generic Name
Kenalog	triamcinolone
Betnelan	betamethasone
Decadron	dexamethasone
Deltacortril	prednisdone
Medrone, Depomedrone	methylprednisolone

Treating Bursitis

Bursitis causes pain in a joint when one of the sacs around tendons or muscles becomes inflamed. When the muscles or tendons move, this inflammation causes pain, in a shoulder, hip, or knee, that is often severe and limiting.

Treatment for bursitis includes temporarily avoiding those movements that cause pain and adding moist heat, rest, and gradually increased exercise. One of the NSAIDs can relieve pain and inflammation. If you still have no improvement, a local injection of a cortisone medication can usually give effective relief.

Treating Tendonitis

Tendonitis happens when a tendon that attaches a muscle to a bone becomes inflamed and causes pain upon use. This common problem can happen at many locations, such as the elbow (tennis elbow, golfer's elbow), shoulder, or foot (Achilles tendon).

To quickly relieve tendonitis, use moist heat, rest, and take an NSAID. In some cases, a local injection of a cortisone medication is used. If there is prolonged pain and the area is important for activity (for a professional athlete, for example), surgery may be necessary to give full recovery.

Hyaluronic Acid Injections for Knee Osteoarthritis (Hyalgan and Synvisc)

Hyaluronic acid injections, a noncortisone medication, are available for osteoarthritis in the knees. Hyaluronic acid is a normal part of joint fluid that helps to make the fluid more elastic and helps protect the cartilage of the joint.

The hyaluronic acid medication is injected directly into the knee each week, usually for three to five consecutive weeks. It's estimated that from 65 to 80 percent of patients find relief, which may last up to six to eight months. Some early studies suggest that continued treatment may slow down the loss of cartilage in the knees. At this time, only the knee is treated with these injections.

These injections are more expensive than cortisone injections, but those who respond may find that the relief lasts much longer than a cortisone injection, thus allowing them to reduce other medications. Side effects are uncommon, but an occasional patient may have a reaction to the medication injected or temporary worsening of joint swelling and pain.

If you use this treatment, continue your usual program of moist heat, exercise, and your medication for treatment of pain and stiffness in other joints. Some arthritis patients get enough relief from these injections to delay other treatments, including surgery. Unfortunately, if the cartilage in your knees is too badly worn, the injections probably won't work.

Commonly Used Nonnarcotic Analgesics

Brand Name	Generic Name
Panadol	paracetamol
Zydol	tramadol
Toradol	ketorolac (NSAID)

Other Pain Medications

Non-narcotic Analgesics

WHAT THEY'RE PRESCRIBED FOR

Sometimes when the combination of moist heat, exercises, paracetamol, and NSAID medication fails to relieve your pain, you might need extra short-term pain relief. This may be at night when pain interferes with sleep or it might happen after extra activity such as a trip to the park with your family, a shopping trip, or when you travel.

The non-narcotic pain medications may act centrally in the brain to change the sensation of pain, yet they have no anti-inflammatory effect. These can be taken safely, remembering that the goal for these medications is occasional relief of pain for a few hours.

POTENTIAL SIDE EFFECTS

With non-narcotic medications, the potential side effects include agitation, anxiety, bloating, gas, constipation, seizures, diarrhea, dizziness, drowsiness, dry mouth, feelings of elation, hallucinations, headache, indigestion, itching, nausea, nervousness, sweating, tremor, vomiting, and weakness.

There is always a chance of dependence with some non-narcotic medications, especially in those patients who have had a dependence problem before. There is a possibility of withdrawal symptoms when discontinuing Zydol (tramadol). A gradual decrease will prevent this from being a major problem.

POSSIBLE INTERACTIONS

Avoid alcohol when taking non-narcotic pain medications. Large doses of Zydol (tramadol) or the combination with drugs such as antidepressants, especially in those who have had seizures in the past, may increase the risk of seizures. Other drug-drug interactions are possible, so check with your doctor before adding Zydol if you're taking any of the following medications: carbamazepine, MAO inhibitors, SSRIs, tricyclic antidepressants, Stelazine, promethazine, quinidine, narcotic pain relievers, sleeping medications (Temazepam, Welldorm, Zopiclone, Zolpidem), or Valium or Diazepam.

Stronger Medications for Chronic Pain

If your joint pain and stiffness are still not well controlled, it's time to check with your doctor to be sure there is no other cause of pain. For example, surgery may be necessary to correct the problem of severe osteoarthritis in the hip or knee. If no other problem is found, then other pain medications are available that allow control of pain and improvement in activity and exercise.

Narcotic Pain Medications

WHAT THEY'RE PRESCRIBED FOR
Narcotic pain relievers work on central nervous system pain receptors to reduce the perception of pain. These medications are available in a wide variety of delivery systems, including patches and liquids, in addition to standard dosage forms. When taken properly, these can be safe and helpful additions to gain control of pain.

Some narcotic pain relievers are short-acting, lasting a few hours and taken only when the pain is severe. If your pain is severe and constant, one of the longer-acting medications can give smooth and continuous relief over many hours. This can help achieve the goal of pain control and also allow an increase in activity. As you improve, the goal is then gradually to lower the dose of narcotic.

These medications must be taken under your doctor's supervision and are closely regulated due to the potential for improper use.

POTENTIAL SIDE EFFECTS
The most common side effects of these medications are sedation, sleepiness, dizziness, and constipation. If you take one of these medications regularly, you may have withdrawal symptoms if you stop suddenly, so follow your doctor's instructions. Higher doses can be dangerous and

may lead to respiratory depression or low blood pressure, and may require emergency treatment.

POSSIBLE INTERACTIONS
Avoid alcohol or sedatives when using these medications. Be sure that your doctor knows you are taking one of these medications before you add any new ones.

Muscle Relaxants

WHAT THEY'RE PRESCRIBED FOR
Muscle relaxants work in the central nervous system to relax skeletal muscles, which can give good relief to those with painful muscle spasms. (These medications may be ineffective unless you are experiencing muscle spasms.)

POTENTIAL SIDE EFFECTS
With muscle relaxants, you may feel dry mouth, dizziness, drowsiness, blurred vision, clumsiness, or unsteadiness. These medications may increase the likelihood of seizures, and older adults sometimes experience confusion and hallucinations. Some muscle relaxants may be habit forming if taken regularly, especially if there are no muscle spasms present.

Commonly Used Narcotic Pain Relievers

Brand Name	Generic Name
Co-codymol	codeine with paracetamol
Darvocet, Wygesic, Coproxamol	dextropropoxyphene with paracetamol
Doloxene	dextropropoxyphene
Duragesic patch	fentanyl, controlled release
Fortral	pentazocine
MS Contin	morphine, controlled release
Oramorph	morphine
Oxycontin	oxycodone, controlled release
Oxynorm	oxycodone
Palladone	hydromorphine
DF118	dihydrocodeine

Commonly Used Muscle Relaxants

Brand Name	Generic Name
Biorphen	orphenadrine citrate
Carisoma	carisoprodol
Lioresal	baclofen
Robaxin	methocarbamol
Skelaxin	metaxalone
Zanaflex	tizanidine

POSSIBLE INTERACTIONS
Muscle relaxants may negatively interact with other drugs such as certain antidepressants like MAO inhibitors; barbiturates, guanethidine, Zydol (tramadol), and central nervous system depressants such as alcohol, narcotics, and tricyclic antidepressants. Talk to your doctor before you add one of these medications.

Tricyclic Antidepressants—Adjunct Analgesics

WHAT THEY'RE PRESCRIBED FOR
Tricyclic antidepressants are older drugs that were originally developed in high doses for depression. For those with fibromyalgia and other types of chronic arthritis pain, tricyclic antidepressants are often used in low doses for pain relief, not depression. These drugs may improve sleep, which causes an increase in endorphins, the body's natural painkiller. They also increase levels of serotonin and norepinephrine in the brain. Patients with chronic arthritis pain often have decreased levels of these calming neurotransmitters. In low doses, these medications do not treat depression. If you have depression, other treatment will be given.

POTENTIAL SIDE EFFECTS
Tricyclic antidepressants may cause drowsiness, dizziness, dry mouth, dry eyes, difficulty in urination and constipation. Older patients are often more sensitive to these side effects, including dizziness and a higher risk of falls.

POSSIBLE INTERACTIONS
These medications may interact with MAO inhibitors, cimetidine, and central nervous system depressants such as alcohol or narcotics.

Pain-Free Arthritis

Commonly Used Tricyclic Antidepressants

Brand Name	Generic Name
Allegron	nortriptyline
Elavil	amitriptyline
Sinequan	doxepin
Tofranil	imipramine

Selective Serotonin Reuptake Inhibitors (SSRIs) and Related Drugs

WHAT THEY'RE PRESCRIBED FOR
SSRIs are mainly used to treat depression, but may also be helpful in the treatment of chronic pain, especially with symptoms of fibromyalgia and osteoarthritis, among others. By blocking the reuptake of serotonin, SSRIs allow more serotonin to travel from neuron to neuron, resulting in improved symptoms.

POTENTIAL SIDE EFFECTS
These medications are usually well tolerated, but you may have side effects such as drowsiness, sweating, nervousness, sexual dysfunction, dry mouth, insomnia, headache, nausea, diarrhea, anorexia, agitation, or weight gain. Some drugs may increase the chance of seizures. Your doctor can help you choose the medication from this group to avoid a specific bothersome side effect.

POSSIBLE INTERACTIONS
SSRIs and related drugs may interact negatively with drugs such as phenytoin, carbamazepine, antipsychotics, benzodiazepines, tryptophan, MAO inhibitors, warfarin, and thioridazine. Talk with your doctor before taking one of these drugs if you are also taking these medications.

Rheumatoid Arthritis and Other Inflammatory Types of Arthritis

So many new medications are available to treat rheumatoid arthritis and other inflammatory types that most rheumatologists now feel confident that patients can achieve excellent control of their pain and stiffness. With many of the medications now available, you can expect a good chance of remission of your arthritis—complete control of pain and

Commonly Used Selective Serotonin Reuptake Inhibitors and Related Drugs

Brand Name	Generic Name
Cipralex	escitalopram
Cipramil	citalopram
Desyrel, Molipixin	trazodone
Effexor	venlafaxine
Prozac	fluoxetine
Seroxat	paroxetine
Serzone	nefazodone
Zispin	mirtazapine
Zyban	bupropion
Lustral	sertraline

stiffness and a noticeable improvement in energy. Most patients say, "I now have my life back."

In rheumatoid arthritis, if you've tried a number of NSAIDs including the COX-2 NSAIDs without good relief, or if you've added prednisone to help more severe pain and stiffness, your doctor will add a second medication. Or, if your X rays show certain changes due to rheumatoid arthritis, the second medication will be added. This second medication is one from the group of disease-modifying drugs (DMARDs). These medications have a good chance of gaining control of joint pain, stiffness, and fatigue while slowing or stopping permanent damage and destruction to the joints. One of the DMARD medications is now started within months after the diagnosis of rheumatoid arthritis when pain and swelling are not very well controlled or X-ray changes are present. It is known that permanent joint damage often begins in the first year of rheumatoid arthritis and that joint damage can be linked to later disability. Since the DMARD medications can stop joint damage, rheumatologists know that the best results happen when the most effective medications are started as early as possible.

Disease-Modifying Drugs (DMARDs)

WHAT THEY'RE PRESCRIBED FOR

Disease-modifying drugs include medications that can be added to gain better control of rheumatoid arthritis and to slow down the progress of the disease. This means it is now possible to stop the destructive changes that can lead to permanent deformities and crippling. About 60 to 80 percent of patients respond to one of these medications and many of those who respond find their arthritis goes into remission. Other medications, including cortisone drugs, may be reduced as well. DMARDs may take up to a few months to work, so it pays to be patient.

The traditional DMARDs in the list below have been used by rheumatologists for many years. They may take three to six months to work and cause side effects serious enough that stopping the medication is common. Unfortunately, these DMARDs often do not produce complete control of pain, swelling, or control of the destructive process in the joints. Methotrexate is the most commonly used of traditional DMARDs. The others are used in combination with methotrexate or alone if methotrexate doesn't work or is not tolerated.

Using methotrexate, the response is often favorable, with up to 40 percent of patients improving in the first month and 75 to 80 percent of patients finding improvement after a few months. This medication is easy to take once weekly in tablet form. Methotrexate is also available as an injection, if the tablets cause nausea. It is most commonly combined with one of the newer biologic DMARDs (see below).

Arava (leflunomide) is a tablet taken daily. This medication may work by limiting the production of T-cells, which can trigger inflammation and joint destruction. It can be given alone and in some cases is combined with methotrexate.

POTENTIAL SIDE EFFECTS
The most common side effects of methotrexate are nausea, mouth sores, rash, abnormal liver tests, hair thinning, and anemia or other blood abnormalities. When the vitamin folic acid is also taken, it can lower the risk of side effects of methotrexate. You should not drink alcohol when you take methotrexate because it raises the risk of liver problems. Your doctor will plan regular blood tests at intervals of one or two months for safety.

When taking Arava (leflunomide), blood tests are taken regularly to monitor for side effects including abnormal liver tests, which may also with methotrexate. Serious liver disease and cirrhosis have been reported, which can usually be avoided by regular blood testing. Occasionally, diarrhea, hair thinning, and mouth sores occur. You should not drink alcohol when taking Arava.

Most Commonly Used Traditional DMARDs

Brand Name	Generic Name
Arava	leflunomide
Matrex	methotrexate
Salazopyrin	sulfasalazine
Plaquenil	hydroxychloroquine

Less Commonly Used Traditional DMARDs

Brand Name	Generic Name
Depen, Cuprimine	penicillamine/distamine
Endoxana	cyclophosphamide
Imuran	azathioprine
Myochrisin	gold sodium thiomalate
Ridaura	auranofin
Neoral	ciclosporin

The Biologic DMARDs

If methotrexate does not give relief, most rheumatologists then add one of the drugs in the list of biologic DMARDs—along with methotrexate. This greatly increases the chances for a good response. Each of these medications when combined with methotrexate may slow down and stop the joint destruction of rheumatoid arthritis—and may help the severe fatigue that often attacks those who suffer from this disease. I believe these are the remarkable benefits of this group of medications.

Biologic DMARDs directly attack cytokines, the chemicals that send messages causing inflammation and joint destruction. The two cytokines that are targeted by the DMARDs now are tumor necrosis factor (TNF) and interleukin 1 (IL-1). Both of these are important producers of joint pain, swelling, and destruction. Newer DMARDs will become available soon.

WHAT THEY'RE PRESCRIBED FOR

Compared to the traditional DMARDs, these new drugs usually have a quicker response, a greater chance of remission of the arthritis pain and swelling, and a higher chance of stopping the permanent damage and

Biologic DMARDs

Brand Name	Generic Name
Enbrel	etanercept
Kineret	anakinra
Remicade	infliximab
Humira	adalimumab

destruction of rheumatoid arthritis. Several medications in this category have tremendous potential for improvement in rheumatoid arthritis:

- *Enbrel*, which is given by self-injection at home twice weekly. Enbrel blocks TNF, which produces inflammation and joint damage. Studies show that Enbrel treatment can actually delay the progress of joint destruction. It is usually given with methotrexate but can be given alone.
- *Remicade*, which is given by intravenous (IV) infusion in the clinic every eight weeks after a series of three infusions given over six weeks. Remicade is an antibody that also blocks TNF, which decreases the chemicals that cause inflammation and joint damage. It is given along with methotrexate.
- *Kineret*, which is an injection given at home daily using a simple injection system. Learning how to self-inject this type of drug has not been a problem with most patients, especially when they realize the potential for improvement. Kineret prevents the action of interleukin, which like TNF can trigger pain, swelling, and joint damage. This medication can be given alone or with methotrexate.
- *Humira* (adalimumab) is given by subcutaneous injection every two weeks. Humira is an antibody that blocks the action of TNF to reduce joint inflammation and damage. It is usually given along with methotrexate.

These medications may give a response within a few weeks to about twelve weeks, and the response usually lasts months or even years. So far, studies show that these medications may slow or stop the progression of the bone destruction in rheumatoid arthritis, a major accomplishment in treatment. They are expensive to develop and manufacture, and their cost is much higher than methotrexate and medications in the first group. There is increasing evidence that higher costs are offset by their ability to prevent permanent damage and expensive surgery and to allow patients to continue to work.

POTENTIAL SIDE EFFECTS

Some possible side effects of these newer medications include sinus infections, reactions in the skin around the site of injection that may last a few days to two weeks, abdominal pain, cough, dizziness, headache, indigestion, other infections, nausea, rash, respiratory problems, sore throat, vomiting, and weakness.

SPECIAL PRECAUTIONS

Tumor necrosis factor plays a major role in the immune system, and blocking TNF's action with these newer DMARDs might lower your resistance to infection. A possible increase in risk of serious infections, particularly tuberculosis, especially in other countries, has been seen in patients taking these medications. Because of this, TB skin testing and chest X ray before starting Remicade or Enbrel is recommended.

If you have a serious infection or suffer from recurrent infections, such as pneumonia, chronic lung disease, or sinus infections, it is usually recommended that you avoid these medications. If you have systemic lupus erythematosus, multiple sclerosis, or congestive heart failure, these medications should not be taken.

Other New Treatments: Prosorba Column

Prosorba column is a treatment that should be considered for severe cases of rheumatoid arthritis that do not respond to treatment with the traditional or biologic DMARDs listed above. In clinical trials, no serious side effects usually occur with this treatment. The effects of the prosorba column may be long lasting, with the average duration of the response up to forty weeks; some responses last as long as seventy-five weeks.

This treatment uses a special column through which blood is treated in a machine and then returned to the donor. Blood is drawn using a method similar to that used during blood donation. The blood is removed through a vein in an arm and treated as it passes through a column. During the treatment, proteins in the blood that produce inflammation are removed and the blood then returned to the body.

Pain-Free Arthritis

Low-Dose Prednisone May Help

In most situations, prednisone is usually avoided, especially in high doses, because of the risk of side effects (explained on page 167). But there are times when rheumatoid arthritis starts or when it has a flare-up that the pain and swelling can severely limit activity. When you must have quick relief and the NSAIDs don't give it, you might consider adding a very low dose of prednisone, such as 5 to 10 milligrams daily. This may give you enough improvement to continue working or doing other activities if not working. This low dose will have minimal side effects, if monitored by your doctor. There is even some evidence that this low dose of prednisone may actually slow down the progress of the joint damage in rheumatoid arthritis when used for the first one to two years.

In our clinics, we consider adding very low doses of prednisone when starting one of the DMARD medications. This is because, at this point, the rheumatoid arthritis is usually severe, but the DMARD may take up to weeks or a few months to begin to work on your rheumatoid arthritis. As the DMARD starts working and your arthritis improves, the prednisone is gradually reduced and stopped.

This short-term use of low-dose prednisone can make a difference in whether you can continue to work or even be independent. If prednisone treatment is continued for more than three months, then another medication can be added to prevent bone loss that can be caused by prolonged prednisone treatment.

Treatment for Gout

An acute gout attack is treated with one of the NSAIDs on page 159. Some that have good results for stopping the acute gout attack are the COX-2 NSAIDs listed on page 166, Indocid (indomethacin), and Voltarol (diclofenac). Usually there is quick relief, within a few days. Colchicine, an older medication, may also be used, but at the high doses required for an acute attack, this medication may have uncomfortable side effects such as nausea or diarrhea. If you still find no relief, your doctor can inject the joint with a cortisone medication, which should stop the attack. If untreated, the attack may last weeks before it subsides.

To prevent future attacks, you must treat the cause, which is an elevated level of uric acid in the blood. This can be treated with allopurinol, a medication that is taken once daily and lowers the body's production of uric acid to decrease its level. If you don't have kidney stones, your doctor might recommend probenecid, a drug that's taken twice daily and increases the body's elimination of uric acid in the urine to lower its level.

While you lower the level of uric acid in the blood to prevent future attacks, it is a good idea also to take a low dose of one of the NSAIDs above or colchicine twice daily for three to six months until the uric acid is lowered below 7.0 mg/dl (milligrams per deciliter). This ongoing therapy will help to prevent gout attacks during this period. Now you can realistically tell yourself "no more gout attacks!" Once the uric acid level has been kept at safe levels, you can stop the NSAID or colchicine and should no longer be bothered by gout as long as you continue allopurinol. (Be sure to review the diet changes necessary to avoid gout on page 65.)

Treating Trigger Finger

Trigger finger (snapping finger) happens when one of the tendons in the palm of the hand that moves a finger slides less easily in one direction and may "catch" or "snap" like a trigger when it moves in one direction. It usually stops the finger in a bent position and causes pain when it is straightened.

The quickest relief for this problem is a local injection of cortisone medication or a minor outpatient surgical procedure. NSAIDs and other oral medications usually do not provide relief.

Treating Lupus

Systemic lupus erythematosus (SLE or lupus) causes arthritis with pain and swelling in many joints, along with fatigue. It may also cause rashes, sun sensitivity, and other problems. Internal organ damage can also occur, most commonly in the kidneys, but can affect the heart, brain, and other organs, too.

If you have this diagnosis, work closely with your doctor. Moist heat, exercise, and rest, along with medications can help control the joint pain and fatigue. Treatment to control kidney and other disease can lead to a normal life expectancy for most patients. It is critical that you follow solid treatment recommendations so you can maximize control of the pain, fatigue, and internal organ damage. Lupus can be an extremely complicated illness, so stay in touch with your doctor as you learn how to manage it.

Treating Ankylosing Spondylitis

Ankylosing spondylitis starts in the lower back and may eventually affect the entire spine with pain and stiffness. If you have this diagnosis, emphasize moist heat and exercises twice daily to keep flexibility and help prevent deformity and loss of function. An NSAID often not only gives excellent relief of the pain and stiffness but allows exercise that is more effective. You may need to try a number of NSAIDs before you find the one that is best for you.

If you don't have luck in finding good relief, other medications are now used in some cases of ankylosing spondylitis to control the disease activity. These include some of the medications used for rheumatoid arthritis, including methotrexate, Enbrel, and other biologic DMARDs. Your doctor can advise you.

Let's Review: 9 Steps to Getting Started with the Latest Medical Treatments

1. Be sure to keep a current and accurate medication record in your Pain-Free Diary, including both prescription and nonprescription medications that you take. The choice of medication depends on the judgment of your doctor. Periodic follow-up is essential to gauge the response to the treatment and to make changes as necessary.
2. Keep accurate records of any natural dietary supplements you take, including herbs, vitamins and minerals, amino acids, glucosamine, or others, and let your doctor know about these.
3. Make an appointment to see your doctor. Put all medications and supplements in a bag and take them with you for your doctor to evaluate.
4. Talk to your doctor about medications listed in this step, and ask if any might be helpful in your situation. If you are prescribed new medication, be sure you fully understand the brand and generic names, doses, reasons for using, and the potential side effects.
5. Make sure all your doctors—your internist, OB-GYN (for women), ophthalmologist, dermatologist, allergist, everyone—know about all the medications you are taking. Before you start another medication for any other condition, ask the prescribing doctor if it may interact with the arthritis medications.

6. Try to use just one pharmacy so your pharmacist can keep accurate records of each medication you take. Sometimes the pharmacist may alert the physician if a patient is using too much of one medication or not enough of another or if there is a potentially dangerous drug-drug interaction.
7. Continue with the twice-daily applications of moist heat and regular exercise for optimal pain relief.
8. Seek help and information from health care professionals but continue to be actively involved in the pain-free process.
9. If you have rheumatoid arthritis, let your doctor know if you want to be proactive with early treatment using DMARDs.

Doctor's Pain-Free Treatment

Your doctor is crucial to good control of your arthritis. However, continue to keep in mind that you are also a vital, active participant in your treatment. The ultimate goal is to control or manage the problem, and only you can accurately follow your physician's recommendations.

Use the guidelines that follow to evaluate your options for pain-free living.

Osteoarthritis

- Use moist heat twice daily, along with the Exercise Treatment (see page 26). Be sure you direct your efforts to maximize the muscle strength and flexibility for your most involved joints, whether the back, knees, hips, or other joints.
- Control your weight. If your arthritis attacks your knees, hips, or back, and you're overweight, start a plan to lose one-half to one pound a week to take the load off your joints.
- Try over-the-counter analgesics or nonsteroidal anti-inflammatory drugs (NSAIDs).
- Add glucosamine (see page 76) at 1,500 mg daily. This dietary supplement may give quick relief for the pain and stiffness and may help slow down the loss of cartilage—the final answer on this is not in yet, but this is a safe medicine if you don't mind paying out-of-pocket for it.
- If over-the-counter paracetamol or ibuprofen doesn't give relief of pain and stiffness, or if either drug loses its effect, a COX-2 NSAID

is usually recommended because of the reduced risk of peptic ulcer disease and bleeding. If your doctor feels you're at low risk for these complications, one of the traditional NSAIDs on page 159 may also work. Find the one that gives you the best relief without side effects.

- For osteoarthritis in the knees, hyaluronic acid injections are available. Surgery may be needed for knees, hips, or other joints.

Fibromyalgia

- Use a warm shower or bath or other moist heat application on the painful trigger points twice daily for 15 minutes each time.
- Start daily stretching and strengthening exercises, as outlined on page 263.
- Slowly add a conditioning exercise daily as on page 19.
- Try one of the NSAIDs on page 159. I find that one of the COX-2 NSAIDs may have a better chance of pain relief in fibromyalgia. At bedtime, add one of the antidepressant medications listed on page 174. You can supplement with nonnarcotic or narcotic pain medications if your doctor feels it's safe.
- Try one or several alternative treatments (see page 66).
- If still no relief, consider evaluation at a comprehensive pain clinic.

Rheumatoid Arthritis

- Apply moist heat to painful joints twice daily. A warm shower or whirlpool spa is an excellent source of moist heat.
- Do the exercises twice daily, along with moist heat baths or applications, as discussed on page 14.
- Find the best NSAID for your pain relief. If a COX-2 NSAID gives relief, there is a lower risk of peptic ulcer and bleeding. You can supplement with pain medications if your doctor so advises.
- If no relief or if your X rays show permanent damage, add one of the DMARD medications on page 177. Remember that early treatment gives better results and can prevent joint damage and disability.
- If still no relief, talk to your doctor about surgical procedures that might help.

PART II

Pain-Free Recipes

Making the right choices in what we eat is a major concern for most of us. Food Marketing Institute (FMI) research shows that more than 70 percent of all shoppers think their diets could be more healthful. The American Dietetic Association (ADA) reports that 60 percent of all consumers are seeking guidelines on choosing healthful foods.

Scientists know more today than ever before about how food can increase or decrease inflammation and pain. For instance, some types of inflammatory arthritis are caused when the immune system goes haywire. It makes good sense to do all you can to keep your immune system functioning at its peak. The mineral zinc helps boost immunity; calcium and magnesium can relax tense muscles. In addition, anti-oxidants, phytochemicals, lycopenes, and a host of vitamins and minerals, such as vitamins A, B_5, B_6, zinc, boron, and copper, are necessary for the production of normal collagen and maintenance of cartilage structures (osteoarthritis affects the cartilage that cushions the ends of bones in your joints). Selenium is vital to reduce the production of inflammatory prostaglandins, the chemicals in the body that cause inflammation, swelling, and pain in arthritis; bioflavonoids help to decrease inflammatory action.

Whether you are a vegetarian, or a meat eater who wants to reduce the amount of meat in your diet, the following Pain-Free Recipes will help to keep your joints strong and pain-free. All recipes are low in fat and calories, and high in healing nutrients for the arthritis patient.

Contents

DRINKS

❖ Fruit Smoothie

Ingredients
1 cup or 140 g fresh or frozen fruit (blueberries, strawberries,
   blackberries, and/or pineapple)
1 medium banana, fresh or frozen
1 cup or 240 ml sweet pineapple juice
2 tablespoons linseed, ground in coffee bean grinder

Directions
Place all ingredients in a blender. Cover and blend till smooth. Pour into
tall glasses and serve.

Yield: Serves 2.

Nutrition information per serving: Calories: 218; Fat: 5 g; Carbohydrates:
44 g; Fiber: 8 g; Protein: 4 g

Hint: If using frozen banana, cut up the banana before it freezes. This will
help you avoid straining your wrist as you cut into frozen fruit.

❖ Green Tea Sangria

Ingredients
3 cups or 710 ml freshly brewed green tea
2 cups or 280 ml fresh blueberries, strawberries, and/or apple slices
1 cup or 240 ml cranberry juice
1 cup or 240 ml pineapple juice
1 cup or 240 ml ginger ale

Directions
Combine all ingredients in a pitcher. Chill and serve.

Yield: Serves 8.

Nutrition information per serving: Calories: 70 g; Fat: 0; Carbohydrates: 13 g; Fiber: 1 g; Protein: 0 g

Hint: Green tea may help to reduce inflammation.

BREADS

❖ Banana Nut Bread

Ingredients
Butter or rapeseed oil for pan
1½ cups or 280 g very ripe bananas, (roughly 3 fruits) mashed
2 eggs
¼ cup or four tablespoons rapeseed oil
⅛ cup or 2 tablespoons honey
2 cups or 250 g wholemeal flour
¼ cup or 4 tablespoons wheat germ
1 teaspoon salt
1 teaspoon baking soda
1 teaspoon vanilla
½ cup or 60 g walnuts, chopped

Directions
Grease a loaf bread pan with butter or rapeseed oil. Mix bananas, eggs, oil, and honey in a medium bowl. Sift flour into a large bowl. Add wheat

germ, salt, and baking soda. Add wet ingredients, including vanilla. Add nuts to mixture. Pour into pan and bake at 180°C/gas mark 4 for 50 minutes. Cook until an inserted toothpick comes out clean. Serve warm with nut butter.

Yield: Makes 10 slices.

Nutrition information per slice: Calories: 206; Fat: 10 g; Carbohydrates: 26 g; Fiber: 4 g; Protein: 6 g

Hint: Use lightweight plastic bowls and lightweight pans to prevent heavy lifting when baking.

❖ Big Fiber Bread

Ingredients
1¼ cups or 300 ml water
2 cups 250 g bread machine flour
1 cup 120 g wholemeal flour
¼ cup or 4 tablespoons wheat bran
2¼ teaspoons active dry yeast
½ cup or 80 g toasted sesame seeds
1 tablespoon milk powder
⅛ cup or 2 tablespoons honey
1 teaspoon salt

Directions
Check bread machine directions and add ingredients accordingly. Serve bread warm, topped with nut butter or jam.

Yield: Serves 10.

Nutrition information per serving: Calories: 216; Fat: 6 g; Carbohydrates: 36 g; Fiber: 4 g; Protein: 7 g

❖ Carrot Cake Muffins

Ingredients
2 cups or 250 g wholemeal flour
½ teaspoon salt
2 teaspoons baking powder
1 cup or 120 g grated carrots
½ cup or 120 ml soy milk
⅓ cup or 80 g rapeseed oil
¼ or 4 tablespoons cup honey
Butter or rapeseed oil for pan

Directions
Sift flour, salt, and baking powder and place in large bowl. Add carrots to dry ingredients and stir. Add soy milk, oil, and honey, and stir thoroughly. Grease muffin pan with butter or rapeseed oil. Fill with batter and bake at 180°C/gas mark 4 for 30 minutes. Muffins are done when inserted toothpick comes out clean.

Yield: Makes 10 muffins.

Nutrition information per serving: Calories: 180; Fat: 8 g; Carbohydrates: 26 g; Fiber: 3 g; Protein: 4 g

Hint: Use spray butter on the muffin tin if buttering the pan hurts your wrists and fingers.

❖ Whole-Wheat Pizza Dough

Ingredients
1 cup or 240 ml warm water
¾ tablespoon dry yeast
½ tablespoon sugar
2 cups or 250 g white flour
1 cup or 120 g wholemeal flour
2 tablespoons olive oil
2 teaspoons salt
1 tablespoon fresh or dried Italian herbs (rosemary, thyme, oregano, basil, etc.)

Directions
Pour water, yeast, and sugar into a mixing bowl. Let stand for 15 minutes. Add flours, olive oil, and salt and stir to combine. Add herbs. Mix until well blended. Place pizza dough on a floured surface and knead until it stretches easily and is smooth to touch. Dough should not be sticky; add water or flour, if necessary. Form dough into a ball and place in a bowl. Cover bowl with plastic wrap and place in a warm, dry place for 30 minutes. Dough should double in size. If desired, knead again and let rise. Roll dough on a floured surface with rolling pin. Spread olive oil in a thin layer over crust. Before placing toppings on pizza, cook at 200°C/gas mark 5 for 3–5 minutes until crust begins to turn a light golden color. After adding toppings, cook at 210°C/gas mark 5 for 5–15 minutes, depending on which toppings you use. Bake until toppings and crust are done.

Yield: Makes 5 servings.

Nutrition information per serving: Calories: 316; Fat: 6 g; Carbohydrates: 57 g; Fiber: 3 g; Protein: 8 g

Hint: Some food processors have a "kneading" option that will help to prevent strain in your fingers and hands while preparing this pizza crust.

SALADS

❖ Delicious Egg Salad with Salmon

Ingredients
6 eggs, boiled and cooled
⅓ cup or 80 g light mayonnaise
2 tablespoons yellow mustard
1 stalk celery, thinly chopped
1 green onion, thinly sliced
3 ounces or 80 g cooked salmon, diced
Salt and pepper to taste
2 tablespoons fresh dill, chopped

Directions
Peel and chop eggs into small pieces. Whisk together mayonnaise and mustard. Add vegetables, salmon, and eggs to the mixture. Mix well and season with salt and pepper. Refrigerate for one hour. Serve topped with fresh dill. This dish is great alone or on a bed of lettuce or sandwich.

Yield: Makes 4 servings.

Nutrition information per serving: Calories: 210; Fat: 15 g; Carbohydrates: 3 g; Fiber: 0 g; Protein: 14 g

Hint: Using canned salmon makes this dish easier to prepare and reduces preparation time.

❖ Saucy Chickpea Salad

Ingredients
1 medium red apple, washed and diced
1 cup or 160 g canned chickpeas, drained and rinsed
1 cup or 160 g canned corn, drained
½ cup or 60 g celery, chopped
1 small red onion, thinly sliced
½ medium cucumber, peeled, thinly sliced
2 tablespoons fresh cilantro, chopped

Dressing
2 tablespoons olive oil
2 tablespoons red wine vinegar
3 tablespoons vegetable stock
1 tablespoon dry mustard
Salt and pepper to taste

Directions
Combine the apple, chickpeas, corn, celery, onion, cucumber, and cilantro in a large bowl. In a small bowl, whisk the dressing ingredients together. Several hours before serving, pour the dressing over the salad and toss well. Refrigerate. Toss the salad again before serving.

Yield: Makes 4 servings.

Nutrition information per serving: Calories: 251 g; Fat: 6 g; Carbohydrates: 43 g; Fiber: 7 g; Protein: 6 g

Hint: Using a lightweight bowl helps protect wrists that are sore or weakened.

❖ Springtime Spinach and Apple Salad

Ingredients
2 large apples
6 cups or 200 g fresh spinach, washed and drained
½ cup or 60 g walnut pieces

Dressing
3 tablespoons olive oil
1 tablespoon balsamic vinegar
Salt and pepper to taste

Directions
Wash, core, peel, and slice apples in thin strips. Toss spinach and apple slices gently in a bowl. Add walnuts and mix. When ready to serve, whisk the dressing ingredients together in a small bowl; pour over salad.

Yield: Makes 6 servings.

Nutrition information per serving: Calories: 159; Fat: 13 g; Carbohydrates: 9 g; Fiber: 3 g; Protein: 5 g

Hint: A salad spinner keeps salad lettuce dry and crisp. It is a great addition to a salad lover's home.

❖ Packed Tuna Salad

Ingredients
⅓ cup or 80 g light mayonnaise
1 tablespoon Dijon mustard

8 ounces or 220 g canned tuna
1 small green onion, thinly chopped
½ apple, peeled, cored, and diced in small squares
2 tablespoons chopped walnuts
½ cup or 60 g celery, thinly chopped
1 cup or 30 g alfalfa sprouts or salad cress
2 cups or 70 g fresh spinach leaves, washed
Salt and pepper to taste

Directions
Place mayonnaise and mustard in a bowl and mix. Add tuna, onion, apple, walnuts, and celery and mix well. When serving, place salad on a bed of spinach and top with alfalfa sprouts or cress.

Yield: Serves 4.

Nutrition information per serving: Calories: 186; Fat: 10 g; Carbohydrates: 7 g; Fiber: 2 g; Protein: 15 g

Hint: Buying packaged spinach leaves will make it easier to prepare this salad. This prevents having to tear off each leaf from the stalk.

❖ Soy Chicken Salad

Ingredients
1 cup or 30 g spinach leaves, washed
2 cups or 60 g red or green leaf lettuce, washed
2 carrots, peeled and sliced into thin rounds
1 cucumber, peeled and diced into small triangles
1 green onion, thinly sliced
1 package soy chicken patties (4 patties)
1 cup or 30 g alfalfa sprouts or salad cress
4 tablespoons linseed, ground in coffee grinder
Honey Mustard Dressing (see recipe below)

Honey Mustard Dressing
4 tablespoons low-fat mayonnaise

1 tablespoon honey
2 tablespoons rapeseed oil
1 teaspoon white vinegar
¼ teaspoon minced onion flakes
1 tablespoon chopped fresh parsley
1 teaspoon yellow mustard

Directions
Place soy chicken patties in oven and cook at 200°C/gas mark 5 for 10 minutes. Chop or tear lettuce into bite-sized pieces. Toss together all other ingredients except alfalfa sprouts and linseed. Mix well. After soy chicken is cooked, allow to cool; chop into small squares. Serve each salad, adding chicken and alfalfa sprouts on top. Sprinkle with ground linseed. Combine all the ingredients for the honey mustard dressing in a separate bowl. Add to each salad to taste.

Yield: Makes 5 servings.

Nutrition information per serving for salad and dressing combined: Calories: 366; Fat: 22 g; Carbohydrates: 29 g; Fiber: 8 g; Protein: 12 g

Hint: Buying prepackaged salad mix prevents having to tear lettuce into bite-sized pieces and speeds up preparation time.

❖ Summer Chicken Salad with Avocado

Ingredients
1½ cups or 290 g brown rice, cooked
2 cups or 280 g chopped, cooked chicken
1 16-ounce or 410 g can of sweet peas, drained
1¼ cups or 150 g sliced celery
½ cup or 80 g green onion, chopped
2 avocados, peeled and cut into ½-inch cubes
2 tablespoons lime juice
2 tablespoons olive oil
Salt, pepper, garlic powder to taste

1 head of cos lettuce
Fresh herbs for garnish: coriander, oregano, or basil
½ cup or 70 g slivered almonds

Directions
Combine rice, chicken, peas, celery, green onion, and avocados in a large bowl and mix gently. Combine lime juice, olive oil, and seasonings in a small bowl and stir well. When ready to eat, pour dressing mixture over rice, chicken, and vegetables. Toss ingredients lightly. Serve over a bed of cos lettuce. Garnish with your favorite fresh herbs and slivered almonds.

Yield: Makes 5 servings.

Nutrition information per serving: Calories: 432; Fat: 23 g; Carbohydrates: 33 g; Fiber: 11 g; Protein: 25 g

SOUPS

✤ Creamy Black Bean Soup

Ingredients
1 tablespoon olive oil
1 cup or 160 g onion, diced
3 cloves garlic, minced
3 green onions, finely chopped
4 cups or 1 liter vegetable stock
1 bay leaf
2 15-ounce or 410 g cans black beans, drained

Directions
Sauté oil, onion, garlic, and green onions in a large pot on medium heat. Cook until onions begin to turn golden. Add beans and vegetable stock to pot. Bring to a boil, adding bay leaf. Simmer for 1 hour. Remove ⅓ cup of black beans. Pour the rest of the soup mixture into a blender and puree. Add blended soup and remaining black beans to pot. Cook an additional 10 minutes, or to taste. Add salt and pepper to taste.

Yield: Makes 5 servings.

Nutrition information per serving: Calories: 205; Fat: 4 g; Carbohydrates: 34 g; Fiber: 14 g; Protein: 11 g

Hint: Use a plastic blender if possible, to prevent strain while lifting.

❖ Savory Green and Red Cabbage Soup

Ingredients
6 cups or 1½ liters vegetable stock
1 pound or 450 g red cabbage, shredded
1 pound or 450 g green cabbage, shredded
3 golden delicious apples, diced
1 large onion, chopped
¼ cup or 4 tablespoons apple cider vinegar
2 tablespoons brown sugar
Salt and pepper to taste
1 cup or 100 g soy cheddar cheese, grated (or regular cheddar cheese)

Directions
In a large soup pot, combine the vegetable stock, cabbages, apples, and onion. Bring the ingredients to a boil. Reduce the heat, cover, and simmer 30 minutes. Stir in the apple cider vinegar and brown sugar. Cook 10 minutes more. Stir in salt and pepper to taste. Top each bowl with a sprinkling of soy cheddar cheese.

Yield: Makes 6 servings.

Nutrition information per serving: Calories: 210; Fat: 7 g; Carbohydrates: 30 g; Fiber: 4 g; Protein: 9 g

Hint: Grated soy cheddar cheese is now available at health food stores and most grocery stores.

❖ Hearty Vegetable Soup

Ingredients
1 tablespoon olive oil
1 small onion, diced
4 medium carrots, peeled and diced
½ red pepper, diced
2 celery stalks, diced
1 yellow squash, diced
2 cloves garlic, chopped
1 bay leaf
2 tablespoons fresh parsley, chopped
Salt and pepper to taste
3 cups or 700 ml vegetable stock
1 cup or 160 g canned chickpeas, drained
1 cup or 170 g canned cannellini or red kidney beans, drained

Directions
Place oil, onion, and vegetables (not including beans) in a large saucepan. Sauté on medium heat 5 minutes, until soft. Add seasonings and continue cooking another 2 minutes. Add enough vegetable stock so that the vegetables are completely covered. Boil mixture, then cover and simmer for 15 minutes. Pour beans into pot and continue cooking another 10 minutes. As soup cooks, you may want to add more water if it is getting too thick.

Yield: Makes 4 servings.

Nutrition information per serving: Calories: 217; Fat: 6 g; Carbohydrates: 30 g; Fiber: 10 g; Protein: 10 g

Hint: Using minced garlic from a jar makes this dish easier and faster to prepare. You can also use frozen carrots and onions.

Pain-Free Arthritis

❖ Split Pea Soup

Ingredients
1 cup or 130 g carrots, chopped
½ cup or 60 g celery, chopped
1 cup or 160 g onion, chopped
1 clove garlic, chopped
1 pound or 450 g raw split green peas
6 cups or 1 liter water
1½ cups or 350 ml vegetable stock
Salt and pepper to taste

Directions
Place chopped vegetables, including garlic, in a pan on medium heat. While the vegetables are cooking, rinse peas and sort, removing any foreign matter. Once onions and carrots start to soften in the pan, add water, vegetable stock, and seasonings. When the water comes to a rolling boil, add peas. Cover and simmer for at least an hour, until peas are soft. Add water to pot, if necessary, as soup cooks.

Yield: Makes 6 servings.

Nutrition information per serving: Calories: 272; Fat: 1 g; Carbohydrates: 49 g; Fiber: 20 g; Protein: 19 g

Hint: If chopping onion is difficult, use a food processor or buy precut onions from the frozen food aisle.

ENTREES

❖ Cordelia's Chicken Purloo

Ingredients
1 large onion, chopped
2 tablespoons olive oil
2 cups or 280 g chicken, cooked and chopped
½ cup or 80 g artichoke hearts, drained and chopped
1 clove garlic, minced

3 cups or 580 g cooked brown rice
1 teaspoon fresh basil
Salt and pepper to taste

Directions
In a heavy pot, sauté onion in olive oil until golden. Stir in cooked chicken, chopped artichoke hearts, and garlic. Add cooked rice, basil, salt and pepper to taste. Heat thoroughly; serve as a side dish or a main dish.

Yield: Makes 4 servings.

Nutrition information per serving: Calories: 356 g; Fat: 11 g; Carbohydrates: 32 g; Fiber: 4 g; Protein: 19 g

Hint: The nutrients in brown rice far outweigh the nutrients in white rice. If you don't like the taste, try mixing half white and half brown rice for your dishes.

❖ Jewel's Pita Pockets

Ingredients
1 garlic clove
1 cup or 70 g red cabbage, shredded
½ celery stalk, coarsely chopped
1 small red onion, coarsely chopped
1 carrot, coarsely chopped
1 cup or 250 g prepared hummus
4 wholegrain pita breads.
½ avocado, sliced thin
½ cucumber, thinly sliced
1 cup or 30 g alfalfa sprouts or salad cress, washed thoroughly
Salt and freshly ground black pepper to taste

Directions
In a blender or food processor put the garlic clove, cabbage, celery stalk, red onion, and carrot. Pulsate several times to shred vegetables. Place vegetables in a bowl and add the hummus. Mix well. Split open the pita bread so it forms a pocket. Spread the hummus mixture evenly on the

inside of the pita bread. Lay the avocado slices on top of the hummus inside the pocket. Lay cucumber slices over the avocado. Sprinkle with sprouts, salt and pepper to taste.

Yield: Makes 4 servings.

Nutrition information per serving: Calories: 343; Fat: 12 g; Carbohydrates: 52 g; Fiber: 11 g; Protein: 13 g

Hint: If you have hip, knee or back pain, gather all food items before you begin to prevent standing for long periods. Also, consider using a stool by the counter if you have problems with back pain when standing for periods of time.

❖ Omelet Pizza

Ingredients
4 frozen soy sausage burger patties
¾ cup or 120 g chopped onion
2 cloves chopped garlic
2 tablespoons olive oil plus extra olive oil for spreading
4 eggs
¼ cup or 4 tablespoons soy milk
1 teaspoon dried oregano
½ teaspoon dried basil
½ recipe Whole-Wheat Pizza Dough (p. 191)
4 ounces or 110 g soy cheddar cheese
Salt and pepper to taste

Directions
Preheat oven to 210°C/gas mark 5. Cook soy sausage burger patties according to package directions. After cooking, crumble the patties. Sauté onion and garlic in olive oil on medium heat until soft. Add crumbled soy sausage and cook until sausage is browned. Whisk eggs and soy milk together and pour the egg mixture into the pan with the other ingredients. Let this cook until the egg mixture becomes firm. While egg is cooking, spread olive oil, oregano, and basil on pizza crust and bake for 5 minutes. Then spread the egg and sausage mixture on pizza crust and

sprinkle soy cheddar cheese on top. Add salt and pepper to taste. Cook at 210°C/gas mark 5 for another 5 minutes, until crust is fully baked.

Yield: Makes 4 servings.

Nutrition information per serving: Calories: 505; Fat: 24 g; Carbohydrates: 46 g; Fiber: 4 g; Protein: 28 g

Hint: Using refrigerated pizza dough, frozen chopped onions, and pre-crumbled soy sausage will help in the preparation of this dish.

❖ Salmon Almondine

Ingredients
¼ cup or 4 tablespoons butter, melted
1 cup or 110 g whole-wheat bread crumbs
¼ cup or 4 tablespoons almonds, finely ground
1 teaspoon lemon juice
Salt and pepper to taste
1 pound or 450 g salmon
2 tablespoons sliced almonds for garnish

Directions
Preheat oven to 200°C/gas mark 5. Combine melted butter, bread crumbs, ground almonds, and lemon juice in a bowl. Stir until well blended. Place fish fillets, skin side down, in a baking dish; cover top of fillets with butter–bread crumb mixture. Sprinkle almond slices over the entire dish. Bake for 25 minutes or until fish is cooked.

Yield: Makes 5 servings.

Nutrition information per serving: Calories: 312; Fat: 20 g; Carbohydrates: 10 g; Fiber: 2 g; Protein: 23 g

Hint: Cold-water fish are the richest source of omega-3 fatty acids, which fight inflammation.

❖ Tasty Tuna Pita

Ingredients
½ tablespoon ginger root, peeled and minced
½ medium onion, chopped coarsely
½ medium cucumber, unpeeled, coarsely chopped
1 apple, unpeeled, cut in quarters
1 tablespoon fresh coriander
12 ounces or 340 g white chunk tuna packed in water, drained and
    chopped
⅓ cup or 80 g light mayonnaise
¼ cup or 4 tablespoons green onion (about 1 large), chopped
Five whole-grain pita breads
5 large pieces of red leaf lettuce, enough to fill pita

Directions
In a blender or food processor, puree ginger, onion, cucumber, apple, and
coriander until well blended. Place blended mixture in a medium bowl.
Add tuna, mayonnaise, and green onion. Cover and refrigerate for 1 hour.
Make a slice around the edge of each pita bread, about one-third of the
circumference. Put the lettuce leaf in the pita and stuff with the tuna
mixture. Serve with fresh vegetables as a side dish.

Yield: Makes 5 servings.

Nutrition information per serving: Calories: 332; Fat: 9 g; Carbohydrates:
42 g; Fiber: 6 g; Protein: 23 g

Hint: Ginger is known to boost digestion and may be helpful in alleviating osteoarthritis pain.

❖ Tex-Mex Tabbouleh

Ingredients
2 cups or 470 ml boiling water
⅔ cup or 125 g uncooked bulgur wheat
1½ tablespoons olive oil
1 cup or 160 g canned sweet corn, rinsed and drained

1 cup or 160 g canned black beans, rinsed and drained
½ cup or 90 g pineapple chunks, diced
1 small red onion, diced
¾ cup or 40 g minced fresh parsley
¾ cup or 40 g minced fresh coriander
¼ cup or 4 tablespoons balsamic vinegar
2 avocados, peel and slice one for the salad, one for garnish
½ teaspoon garlic powder
Salt and pepper to taste

Directions
In a large pot, combine boiling water and bulgur. Stir well and let stand for 1 hour. Stir occasionally. Drain any remaining liquid. Use ½ tablespoon oil to grease a cookie sheet. Place the corn on the cookie sheet and broil until light golden. Add cooked bulgur wheat to a large bowl. Stir in the corn, black beans, pineapple, onion, parsley, coriander, 1 tablespoon olive oil, and balsamic vinegar. Peel and slice 1 avocado and stir into the bulgur mixture. Add spices to taste. Toss well. Put the bulgur mixture on a large platter and garnish with remaining avocado slices just before serving.

Yield: Makes 6 servings.

Nutrition information per serving: Calories: 309; Fat: 15 g; Carbohydrates: 43 g; Fiber: 12 g; Protein: 8 g

Hint: Using spray oil on the cookie sheet will ease the pain of oiling the pan.

❖ Wholesome Veggie Pizza

Ingredients
Whole-Wheat Pizza Dough (see page 191)
1¼ cups or 125 g soy mozzarella cheese, shredded
1½ cups or 180 g of your favorite vegetables (broccoli, onions, spinach, etc.), chopped
1 teaspoon garlic powder
1 teaspoon Italian seasonings
¼ teaspoon salt
¼ teaspoon pepper

Directions
Preheat oven to 220°C/gas mark 6 Lightly grease a pizza pan or pizza stone. Place in oven so pan or stone gets hot. Prepare the Whole-wheat Pizza Dough. When dough is ready, roll onto the warm pan. Cover the crust with ¼ cup of the soy cheese and press gently into the crust to within an inch of the edge, leaving room for the crust. Top with your vegetables. Sprinkle the rest of the cheese over the vegetables and seasonings, if desired. Bake for 10–20 minutes, until the crust is golden and the cheese is bubbling. Oven temperatures vary in different ovens; watch your pizza to determine when your crust and vegetables are ready. Let the pizza cool slightly on a rack before serving.

Yield: Makes 5 servings.

Nutrition information per serving: Calories: 484; Fat: 16 g; Carbohydrates: 65 g; Fiber: 4 g; Protein: 21 g

Hint: Using refrigerated pizza dough will make preparing this dish easier on your hands and wrists.

❖ Tempeh Fajitas

Ingredients
8 ounces or 220 g tempeh, sliced into ¼-inch by ½-inch squares
2 tablespoons soy sauce
1 clove garlic, minced
¼ teaspoon cumin
1 tablespoon rapeseed oil
1 onion, sliced in strips
1 cup or 70 g broccoli, diced
1 cup or 70 g portabello mushrooms, sliced in strips
8 6-inch whole-wheat tortillas, warmed
½ cup or 50 g soy cheese, shredded
½ recipe of Quick Guacamole (p. 217)

Directions
Marinate tempeh in soy sauce, garlic, and cumin for 2 hours, spooning marinade over tempeh from time to time. After marinating, sauté

tempeh in oil on medium-high heat for 5 minutes, stirring throughout. Add onion and broccoli to mixture and cook until vegetables soften. Add mushrooms and sauté, stirring throughout, until all ingredients are cooked. For each serving, have each person top their tortilla with the tempeh-vegetable mixture, soy cheese, and guacamole to their liking. After adding toppings, roll up tortillas and eat.

Yield: Makes 4 servings.

Nutrition information per serving: Calories: 509; Fat: 25 g; Carbohydrates: 47 g; Fiber: 9 g; Protein: 23 g

Hint: Tempeh has all the benefits of soy and tastes great, too, with a meaty, firm texture. You can find it in health food stores and most grocery stores.

❖ Tanner's Polynesian Tofu Baguette

Ingredients
14 ounces or 400 g firm tofu
⅛ teaspoon salt
⅛ teaspoon pepper
1 tablespoon olive oil
½ cup or 80 g chopped onion
4 wholegrain baguette rolls or 8 thick slices of wholegrain bread

Polynesian sauce
8 ounces or 220 g unsweetened crushed pineapple
1 tablespoon fresh ginger, peeled and grated
1 tablespoon cider vinegar
6½ ounces or 180 g plum sauce

Directions
Cut tofu into ½-inch slices. Wrap slices in paper towels to absorb the liquid (takes about 30 minutes). Prepare the sauce while the tofu is draining. Add the pineapple with liquid, grated ginger, vinegar, and plum sauce in a small saucepan; bring to a boil. Cook for 1 minute. Remove from heat; set aside.

Sprinkle the tofu slices with salt and pepper. Heat the olive oil in a large frying pan over medium-high heat. Add tofu; cook for several minutes, turning to brown each side. Add onion and sauté until soft. Brush the Polynesian sauce over tofu, and cook 2 minutes. Turn slices over and brush again to allow the sauce to glaze the tofu. Evenly distribute the tofu slices on the baguettes and top with a little sauce.

Yield: Makes 4 servings.

Nutrition information per serving: Calories: 470; Fat: 14 g; Carbohydrates: 68 g; Fiber: 6 g; Protein: 19 g

Hint: Use pineapple frequently since the natural enzymes help to decrease inflammation.

❖ Red Wine Chicken

Ingredients
1 cup or 240 ml red wine
1 tablespoon fresh parsley, chopped
1 clove garlic, thinly sliced
4 whole boneless chicken breasts, skin removed
1 tablespoon garlic powder

Directions
Combine red wine, parsley, and garlic in a bowl. Place chicken, which may be divided in half, in the marinade and let sit, refrigerated, for at least 3 hours, spooning marinade over chicken every half-hour. Then rub garlic powder over chicken. Place in an oiled frying pan and sauté chicken on medium-high heat. Sauté chicken until fully cooked, turning once.

Yield: Makes 4 servings (or 8 half-breast servings).

Nutrition information per serving: Calories: 300; Fat: 3 g; Carbohydrates: 1 g; Fiber: 0 g; Protein: 54 g

Hint: Studies have found that red wine reduces the pain, swelling, and discomfort of arthritis. However, use in moderation.

❖ Lucy's Baked Fish

Ingredients
1 pound or 450 g fish fillets (tuna or salmon)
1 tablespoon lemon juice

Marinade
½ teaspoon salt
⅛ teaspoon fresh grated ginger
½ teaspoon cumin powder
3 garlic cloves, chopped
3 tablespoons fresh parsley, chopped

Directions
Place fish in a large bowl and coat with the marinade. Cover and marinate for 1 hour in the refrigerator, turning frequently to marinate entire fish. Coat a baking dish with nonstick cooking spray. Place the fish in the dish and cover with marinade. Bake uncovered at 400°F for 25 minutes or until cooked through. Sprinkle with lemon juice.

Yield: Makes 5 servings.

Nutrition information per serving: Calories: 138; Fat: 5 g; Carbohydrates: 1 g; Fiber: 0 g; Protein: 22 g

Hint: Both tuna and salmon are high in omega-3 fatty acids. Studies show that omega-3s help to decrease inflammation.

❖ Grilled Pesto Chicken Sandwich

Ingredients
1 tablespoon olive oil
2 wholegrain baguettes or 4 slices thickly sliced wholegrain bread
Authentic Pesto (recipe follows)
1 cup or 140 g cooked chicken, shredded
½ cup or 20 g spinach, washed and cut into strips

Directions
Spread ¼ tablespoon oil on one side of each slice of bread. Divide pesto into quarters, spreading a quarter of the pesto on the other side of each slice of bread. Place chicken in the middle of the bread, between the pesto sides. Grill sandwiches, oil sides down, on hot griddle until warmed and golden brown, flipping once. Stuff sandwiches with fresh spinach. Cut each sandwich in half and serve.

Authentic pesto
1 large clove garlic
1 cup or 30 g fresh basil leaves
1½ tablespoons pine nuts
2 tablespoons olive oil
Salt and pepper to taste

Directions
Blend ingredients in a food processor or blender.

Yield: Makes 2 servings.

Nutrition information per serving: Calories: 510; Fat: 29 g; Carbohydrates: 32 g; Fiber: 5 g; Protein: 26 g

Hint: Animal protein may increase inflammation. Try substituting with soy products or fish when possible.

PASTA/GRAINS/RICE

❖ Beans and Greens with Quinoa

Ingredients
1 cup or 200 g quinoa plus 2½ cups water for cooking
1 onion, chopped
1 clove garlic, finely chopped
2 tablespoons olive oil
2 tablespoons red wine vinegar
2 tablespoons water

8 cups or 260 g of greens (kale, collard, chard, or turnip greens)
2 cups or 340 g black-eyed peas, drained
Salt and pepper to taste

Directions
Rinse quinoa and sort to remove any foreign matter. Place quinoa in 2½ cups boiling water; cover, and simmer for 15 minutes or until quinoa is soft and water is absorbed. While quinoa is cooking, sauté onion and garlic in olive oil until onion softens. Add greens and vinegar to the pot. Add 2 tablespoons of water if necessary. Cook on medium-low heat until greens are wilted. Then add the black-eyed peas and heat until warm. Serve beans and greens over quinoa.

Yield: Makes 4 servings.

Nutrition information per serving: Calories: 330; Fat: 10 g; Carbohydrates: 50 g; Fiber: 6 g; Protein: 12 g

Hint: Dark leafy green vegetables are powerful sources of nutrients. This dish supplies a high amount of iron, calcium, and fiber from vegetable sources.

❖ Paella with Loads of Veggies

Ingredients
1 large red onion, peeled and sliced
2 tablespoons olive oil
1 teaspoon garlic powder
2 cups or 400 g long-grain rice, uncooked
4 cups or 950 ml vegetable stock
1 cup or 120 g artichoke hearts
1 cup or 160 g broccoli florets
1 cup or 140 g frozen small peas
3 large carrots, sliced
Salt and pepper to taste
4 bay leaves
½ teaspoon thyme
1 teaspoon onion powder

Directions
In a large frying pan, sauté the onion in the olive oil. Add garlic powder. Stir in rice and brown lightly. Add vegetable stock. Add artichoke hearts, broccoli florets, peas, and carrots. Cover and reduce heat to simmer for 10 minutes. Stir in salt, pepper, bay leaves, thyme, and onion powder. Cover and continue to simmer for 10 to 15 minutes or until rice is done. The liquid should be absorbed but the rice should still be moist.

Yield: Makes 4 servings.

Nutrition information per serving: Calories: 295; Fat: 6 g; Carbohydrates: 50 g; Fiber: 10 g; Protein: 9 g

Hint: When you cook, double or triple the recipe and make "batches" of the dish. You can freeze individual portions or enough for a family meal. Pull out the batch when you don't have the energy to cook or your arthritis is flaring up and you need a break from preparing a meal.

❖ Sesame Couscous with Chickpeas

Ingredients
2 cups or 470 ml vegetable stock
1½ cups or 260 g couscous
1 tablespoon olive oil
2 cups or 140 g broccoli florets, chopped in large bite-sized pieces
1 medium onion, chopped
15 ounces or 410 g tinned chickpeas, drained
¼ cup or 4 tablespoons sesame seeds
Salt and pepper to taste

Directions
Pour vegetable stock into a medium saucepan. Bring to a boil. Stir in the couscous with a fork, cover, and let the water absorb for about 12–15 minutes. In a frying pan, heat the olive oil. Sauté the broccoli and onion for 2–3 minutes on medium heat. Cover the vegetables and cook on low until vegetables are tender (3–4 minutes). Stir in the chickpeas and cover the pan; heat for 3–4 minutes longer. Set aside. In a large serving bowl,

add vegetable mixture to couscous. Stir in sesame seeds. Add salt and pepper to taste and serve.

Yield: Makes 5 servings.

Nutrition information per serving: Calories: 396; Fat: 8 g; Carbohydrates: 68 g; Fiber: 9 g; Protein: 14 g

Hint: Broccoli helps the body utilize calcium, as it is loaded with calcium and magnesium. This is beneficial for people suffering from rheumatoid arthritis.

✢ Caesar Pasta with Prawns

Ingredients
12 ounces or 340 g wholemeal pasta
3 cups or 210 g fresh broccoli, washed and chopped in bite-size pieces
½ cup or 120 ml prepared Caesar salad dressing
12 ounces or 340 g fresh prawns, peeled and deveined

Directions
Boil pasta according to package directions. About 3 minutes before pasta is ready, add broccoli to boiling water. Drain pasta and broccoli. In a large frying pan, heat 2 tablespoons of the Caesar dressing over medium-high heat. Add prawns and stir-fry 3–4 minutes or until prawns are pink and cooked through. Drain pasta and broccoli; transfer to a serving bowl. Toss in remaining dressing and prawns.

Yield: Makes 6 servings.

Nutrition information per serving: Calories: 352; Fat: 10 g; Carbohydrates: 46 g; Fiber: 6 g; Protein: 21 g

Hint: Use a strainer in your pot when cooking the pasta. The pasta can be lifted out easier than lifting the whole pot of boiling water. Have a large bowl next to your stovetop. Lift the pasta into the bowl and carry it to the sink to drain.

❖ Sassy Pasta

Ingredients
12 ounces or 340 g wholemeal pasta (fettuccine, linguine, or angel hair)
3 cups or 210 g broccoli florets
3 whole carrots, thinly sliced
2 tablespoons olive oil
2 medium courgettes, thinly sliced
12 ounces or 340 g canned white tuna, packed in water
Salt and pepper to taste

Pesto sauce
2 cups or 70 g fresh basil leaves
⅓ cup or 40 g pine nuts
1 clove garlic
1 tablespoon olive oil
Salt and pepper to taste

Directions
Boil a large pot of water; cook pasta until al dente, then drain. While pasta is cooking, combine pesto ingredients in a food processor and blend. Add more olive oil if pesto is too chunky or difficult to blend. Set aside.

Steam broccoli and carrots until crisp-tender. Add 2 tablespoons oil to a frying pan, add courgettes, and stir until courgettes start to turn golden. Add pesto sauce to pasta, and toss. Add cooked vegetables and tuna. Add salt and pepper to taste.

Yield: Makes 6 servings.

Nutrition information per serving: Calories: 413; Fat: 11 g; Carbohydrates: 52 g; Fiber: 9 g; Protein: 26 g

❖ Spicy Tempeh with Spinach

Ingredients
12 ounces or 340 g tempeh, chopped in thick squares
2 tablespoons oil
4 cloves garlic, chopped

½ onion, finely chopped
2–4 tablespoons soy sauce
6 cups or 200 g fresh spinach, washed and chopped
Salt and pepper to taste

Directions
Place tempeh in pan with oil and 2 cloves of garlic. Sauté for 2 minutes, then cover and steam for 3 minutes. Remove lid and add onion to pan. Cook an additional 5 minutes or until onion is soft and golden. Add the soy sauce, remaining garlic, and spinach and sauté for 2–3 minutes or until spinach is wilted. Serve over rice noodles or pasta for an Asian-style noodle dish.

Yield: Makes 4 servings.

Nutrition information per serving: Calories: 149; Fat: 10 g; Carbohydrates: 8 g; Fiber: 4 g; Protein: 9 g

Hint: If unloading the dishwasher daily aggravates your arthritis symptoms, consider using dishes from the dishwasher instead of having to unload them and later pull them from the shelf.

VEGETABLES

❖ Avocado-Alfalfa Roll-Ups

Ingredients
4 6-inch whole-wheat tortillas
1 cup or 250 g prepared hummus
1 avocado, thinly sliced
½ cucumber, peeled and very thinly sliced
1 cup or 30 g alfalfa sprouts or salad cress
1 medium carrot, grated
Salt and pepper to taste

Directions
Spread the tortillas on a tray. Divide toppings and vegetables into quarters. Spread a quarter of the prepared hummus on the tortillas and

spread evenly. Put the avocado slices on top of the hummus, down the center. Lay cucumber slices over the avocado slices. Place a quarter of the alfalfa sprouts and carrots over the avocado. Add salt and pepper to taste. Tightly roll the tortilla to create a log shape. Use toothpicks to hold the roll-up together. Wrap the roll tightly in plastic wrap and refrigerate for several hours. Cut the wrap in half crosswise on a slight diagonal.

Yield: Makes 4 servings.

Nutrition information per serving: Calories: 300; Fat: 16 g; Carbohydrates: 30 g; Fiber: 9 g; Protein: 10 g

Hint: Hummus is a great way to get protein without having to eat meat. There are many different types of hummus on the market today.

❖ Easy Kale

Ingredients
4 cups or 130 g kale
1 tablespoon rapeseed oil
2 tablespoons water
1 tablespoon brown sugar
Salt and pepper to taste

Directions
Wash kale, and remove the leaves from the thick stalks. Chop leaves in small strips. Place greens and oil in 2 tablespoons of water in a large saucepan and sauté. Cook 3–5 minutes until greens wilt. Add the brown sugar, stir, and mix well.

Yield: Makes 4 servings.

Nutrition information per serving: Calories: 56; Fat: 3 g; Carbohydrates: 5 g; Fiber: 1 g; Protein: 1 g

Hint: Rapeseed, soybean, and olive oil are healthy sources of cooking oil as they have the best proportion of omega-3s, -6s, and -9s.

❖ Herbed Carrots

Ingredients
2 cups or 260 g baby carrots, washed
1 tablespoon butter
2 tablespoons slivered almonds
1 teaspoon coriander
1 teaspoon fresh chives, chopped
Juice from ½ lemon
Salt and pepper to taste

Directions
Steam carrots and drain. Melt butter in a pan and add almonds and coriander. Cook on medium heat for 2 minutes. Add carrots, chives, and lemon juice to the mix and continue to cook until all ingredients are warmed. Serve immediately.

Yield: Makes 2 servings.

Nutrition information per serving: Calories: 122; Fat: 10 g; Carbohydrates: 7 g; Fiber: 2 g; Protein: 2 g

Hint: You should aim to get at least 9,000 IU of beta-carotene daily to keep your immune system strong. One large carrot provides 20,000 IU of beta-carotene.

❖ Quick Guacamole

Ingredients
2 large avocados, pitted
1 teaspoon garlic powder
½ teaspoon salt
1 tablespoon lime juice

Directions
Mash avocados and add seasoning. Cover and refrigerate for 1 hour, then serve.

Yield: Makes 5 servings.

Nutrition information per serving: Calories: 132; Fat: 12 g; Carbohydrates: 6 g; Fiber: 4 g; Protein: 2 g

Hint: Avocado is loaded with B$_6$, an essential B vitamin.

❖ Spinich with Apple and Pine Nuts

Ingredients
1 medium onion, sliced
1 tablespoon extra virgin olive oil
1 large bunch or 80 g spinach, washed
½ tablespoon garlic powder
¼ teaspoon pepper
¼ cup or 4 tablespoons vegetable stock
1 apple, chopped into small squares
4 tablespoons lightly toasted pine nuts

Directions
Sauté onion in oil over low to medium heat, stirring often for 3–4 minutes. Tear spinach leaves off the stems and cut into small strips. Add the spinach, garlic powder, pepper, and stock to the pan. Cover and cook for 2–5 minutes more, or until greens are tender enough to chew. Remove from heat. Add apple and pine nuts. Cover and simmer for a few minutes more to allow apples to soften a bit.

Yield: Makes 4 servings.

Nutrition information per serving: Calories: 117; Fat: 8 g; Carbohydrates: 11 g; Fiber: 3 g; Protein: 3 g

Hint: This dish is loaded with ingredients that help fight inflammation and add necessary nutrients to the diet including onion, leafy greens, garlic, olive oil, and apple.

✤ Vegetarian Pâté

Ingredients
2 tablespoons olive oil
½ cup or 80 g onion, diced
2 cups or 270 g canned green beans, drained
½ cup or 120 g light mayonnaise
¼ cup or four tablespoons walnuts, chopped
2 tablespoons white wine (optional)

Directions
Pour olive oil into small pan and sauté onion on medium heat until just golden. Place all ingredients in food processor and blend until smooth. Chill. Serve with toasted whole-wheat pita bread or fresh raw vegetables.

Yield: Makes 8 servings.

Nutrition information per serving: Calories: 112; Fat: 11 g; Carbohydrates: 3 g; Fiber: 1 g; Protein: 1 g

Hint: Walnuts are a great source of omega-3. English walnuts have a higher concentration of omega-3 than black walnuts.

✤ Barbecued Tofu

Ingredients
8 ounces or 220 g firm tofu, cut ½ inch thick, in rectangles
1 tablespoon olive oil
1 tablespoon honey
3 tablespoons barbecue sauce
1 teaspoon garlic powder

Directions
Cut tofu and place in olive oil in a pan on medium heat. Sauté for about 5 minutes, then pour honey, barbecue sauce, and garlic powder on top. Flip tofu and sauté for 3–5 minutes more. Serve as a main dish or side dish. This dish is great with Easy Kale (see page 216).

Yield: Makes 2 servings.

Nutrition information per serving: Calories: 234; Fat: 11 g; Carbohydrates: 17 g; Fiber: 3 g; Protein: 20 g

Hint: You can make several servings of this and refrigerate what you don't eat. It makes great leftovers.

✢ Gingered Veggies

Ingredients
1 head cabbage, shredded
3 cups or 210 g broccoli, chopped into bite-size pieces
4 carrots, peeled and chopped in thin strips
1 onion, sliced into thin rings
2 tablespoons olive oil
3 tablespoons low-sodium soy sauce
2 cloves garlic, minced
2–3 tablespoons fresh ginger, peeled and grated
½ teaspoon garlic powder
½ teaspoon onion powder
Salt and pepper to taste

Directions
Heat a large wok or frying pan to medium-high heat and add olive oil and vegetables, including garlic and ginger. Sauté until vegetables are crisp-tender. Add seasonings and serve.

Yield: Makes 6 servings.

Nutrition information per serving: Calories: 126; Fat: 5 g; Carbohydrates: 19 g; Fiber: 7 g; Protein: 5 g

✤ Asian Coleslaw

Ingredients
3 cups or 210 g purple cabbage, grated
3 cups or 210 g green cabbage, grated
1 onion, halved
3 celery stalks, diced
4 carrots, diced
1 tablespoon ginger, minced
2 cups or 470 ml water
1 tablespoon honey
½ cup or 120 ml balsamic vinegar
1 tablespoon horseradish
¼ cup or 4 tablespoons light mayonnaise
Salt to taste

Directions
Grate the cabbages into a large bowl. In a blender place 1 cup of the grated cabbage, the onion, celery, carrots, ginger, and 2 cups water. Process until chunky. Drain, pressing the water out of the mixture. In a small bowl add the blended mixture and the honey, vinegar, horseradish, and mayonnaise. Stir this mixture and pour over the grated cabbage in the bowl. Add salt to taste. Let the slaw marinate for several hours, spooning the dressing over the cabbage several times.

Yield: Makes 8 servings.

Nutrition information per serving: Calories: 81; Fat: 2 g; Carbohydrates: 15 g; Fiber: 3 g; Protein: 2 g

❖ Retro Seven-Layer Dip

Ingredients
1 Quick Guacamole (p. 217) or prepared guacamole
½ recipe Vegetarian Refried Beans (p. 223) or 2 cups or 480 g canned
    refried beans
½ cup or 30 g shredded lettuce
4 green onions, chopped
½ cup or 60 g black olives, sliced
1 cup or 100 g shredded soy cheese
2 tablespoons coriander, fresh and chopped

Directions
Prepare Quick Guacamole and Vegetarian Refried Beans (you can also used canned beans if you prefer). In a 9-inch pan spread the refried beans. Pour guacamole over the refried beans. Add shredded lettuce, green onions, and black olives. Top with the soy cheese. Sprinkle chopped coriander over the dip, cover, and refrigerate until serving. This dip is great with your favourite vegetables, whole-wheat pita bread, or corn chips.

Yield: Makes 10 servings.

Nutrition information per serving: Calories: 191; Fat: 12 g; Carbohydrates: 14 g; Fiber: 5 g; Protein: 8 g

Hint: Avoid high-fat dairy products when possible. Try using the new soy- and rice-based cheeses for low-fat alternatives. Some people find that diary products aggravate arthritis and pain.

❖ The Simple Soybean

Ingredients
2 cups or 450 g green soybeans (otherwise known as edamame, usually
    available in the UK in Chinese grocery stores)
¼ teaspoon salt
¼ teaspoon garlic powder
½ teaspoon onion powder

Directions
In a large pot, bring 6 cups or 1½ liters of water to a boil. Add soybeans and return to a boil. Cook the soybeans for 15 minutes. Drain well and add spices. Shell pods before eating.

Yield: Makes 4 servings.

Nutrition information per serving: Calories: 188; Fat: 9 g; Carbohydrates: 14 g; Fiber: 5 g; Protein: 16 g

Hint: Edamame is very popular in Japanese cooking. The soybeans taste like boiled peanuts and are a healthy side dish or snack.

❖ Vegetarian Refried Beans

Ingredients
1 small onion, chopped
2 cloves chopped garlic
2 tablespoons olive oil
30 ounces or 410 g canned red kidney beans
2 cups or 470 ml vegetable stock
Salt and pepper to taste
2 tablespoons fresh coriander, chopped (optional)

Directions
Sauté onion and garlic in olive oil on medium heat until onions soften. Add half the beans and half the stock to the pan. Continue cooking the mixture and mash beans with the back of a fork while cooking. Add the rest of the beans and stock and continue mashing the beans. Cook and mash until the beans are soft and all the liquid is absorbed. Add salt and pepper to taste. Serve garnished with fresh coriander.

Yield: Makes 6 servings.

Nutrition information per serving: Calories: 183; Fat: 6 g; Carbohydrates: 26 g; Fiber: 8 g; Protein: 9 g

Hint: If mashing the beans with a fork is difficult, try processing in a blender or a food processor.

DESSERTS

✤ Apple-Blueberry Sauce

Ingredients
2 medium-tart apples, chopped into large chunks
140 g cup fresh blueberries
2 tablespoons sugar
¾ cup or 180 ml water
1 teaspoon cinnamon
½ teaspoon nutmeg
1 teaspoon cornflour
¼ teaspoon lemon juice
Pinch of salt

Directions
Combine all ingredients and stir well. Add to saucepan on medium-high heat and bring mixture to a boil. Lower heat and simmer until mixture thickens and fruits are soft. If necessary, add water to desired consistency. The sauce should be watery enough to pour over whole-wheat pancakes.

Yield: Makes 6 servings.

Nutrition information per serving: Calories: 62; Fat: 0 g; Carbohydrates: 16 g; Fiber: 2 g; Protein: 0 g

Hint: You can also sprinkle flaxseeds over pancakes and the apple-blueberry sauce for extra essential fatty acids. Invest in a coffee bean grinder and grind the flaxseeds until they are very fine for ease in digestion.

✤ Samba's Vanilla Bean Boats

Ingredients
3 small or 1½ large papayas
2 vanilla beans
½ cup or 120 ml coconut milk
½ cup or 70 g sliced almonds

1 lime (decoration)
Tropical flowers (decoration)

Directions
Preheat oven to 190°C/gas mark 4. Cut the papayas into 6 servings and scoop out the seeds. Place the pieces of papaya on a baking sheet. Straighten the vanilla beans on a cutting board and cut lengthwise into ¾-inch strips. Split the beans open, and scrape a few seeds into each papaya half. Put the beans in the papaya pieces and pour some coconut milk over the fruit. Cover the papaya boats with foil. Bake for 10–15 minutes or until heated through. On a large platter place the 6 boats decorated with almond slices, thin slices of lime, tropical flowers if available, or flowers from your garden (washed), and serve.

Yield: Makes 6 servings.

Nutrition information per serving: Calories: 150; Fat: 9 g; Carbohydrates: 17 g; Fiber: 4 g; Protein: 3 g

Hint: One ounce of almonds has 7 mg of vitamin E, which may be beneficial to those suffering with arthritis.

❖ Baked Apples

Ingredients
2 apples (Granny Smiths work best)
¼ cup or 4 tablespoons raisins
2 tablespoons honey
¼ teaspoon cinnamon
2 teaspoons lemon juice
½–1 cup or 120–240 ml water (for bottom of pan)

Directions
Grease small pan with butter. Wash and core apples and place in pan. After coring, use a knife to scoop out a little "bowl" in the middle of the apples. Divide raisins, honey, and cinnamon evenly and place ingredients in the "bowls" of the apples. Add lemon juice to the water and pour

liquid into the bottom of the pan, around apples. Bake at 190°C/gas mark 4 for 15 minutes. Every 5 minutes, pour the lemon-water mixture over the tops and sides of the apples until coated.

Yield: Makes 4 servings.

Nutrition information per serving: Calories: 100; Fat: 0 g; Carbohydrates: 27 g; Fiber: 2 g; Protein: 0 g

Hint: Invest in an apple corer to make this dish easier and less painful to prepare.

❖ Tropical Fruit Platter

Ingredients
1 pineapple
1 mango
1 small or ½ large papaya
2 kiwi
2 cups or 340 g of seasonal melon, cantaloupe or honeydew

Directions
Peel pineapple and slice into ½-inch-thick rings. Peel mango and cut off fruit from the stone. Slice into long strips. Peel papaya and dice into desired bite-size pieces. Peel kiwi and slice into ½-inch-thick rings. Using a melon ball scoop, cut the melon into round balls. Place the pineapple slices decoratively in a ring around the edge of the large platter. Then place a layer of mango on top of the pineapple, more toward the center. Continue layering the fruit until it is all on the platter. Stack melon balls in the center of the fruit ring.

Yield: Serves 4.

Nutrition information per serving: Calories: 165; Fat: 1 g; Carbohydrates: 41 g; Fiber: 5 g; Protein: 3 g

Hint: This fruit platter combines the best fruits for arthritis pain: papaya and mango are full of vitamin E and beta-carotene, and cantaloupe has a high amount of beta-carotene as well.

PART III

Special Situations

For most cases of arthritis, the Pain-Free Program will work fast to ease symptoms and let you reclaim an active life again. If carefully followed, you should begin to experience a reduction of pain, inflammation, stiffness, and other symptoms in just a few weeks.

Yet, there are still those special situations where this multifaceted program may not bring optimal relief. For instance, if you have combination cases of arthritis, you may need a more specialized program to end pain, including specific medications for each type of arthritis. Or if you are contemplating starting a family, you'll need to work closely with your rheumatologist from before conception until after delivery to make sure your arthritis flares are kept to a minimum, and there is no worsening of the disease or harm to the fetus. In some cases, you might need a surgical procedure to alleviate pain and stiffness.

In Special Situations, you'll find helpful information for these and other unique circumstances. As you read this section, I urge you to continue using your Pain-Free Diary to jot down personal concerns, questions about treatment, or new ideas to share with your doctor.

Combination Cases

Some people are unaware that you can have two or more types of arthritis at the same time. On the other hand, you can have arthritis and another pain-related ailment such as carpal tunnel syndrome, TMJ, or bursitis. For example, I treat many patients who have rheumatoid arthritis and fibromyalgia. Other patients have osteoarthritis and rheumatoid arthritis or osteoarthritis and gout. A few patients have rheumatoid arthritis, fibromyalgia, carpal tunnel syndrome, and back pain from disc disease or osteoporosis. The pain combinations often seem endless!

No matter how complicated your arthritis seems, getting a proper diagnosis is the best way to get the most effective treatment for each type of arthritis. The best time to consider discussing an evaluation with your doctor is when your arthritis symptoms change or when you lose control of the pain and stiffness.

Here is the rule of thumb I give to my patients: If at any time your arthritis suddenly worsens, behaves differently, or loses the response to medications, call the clinic and make an appointment to see a doctor. In some cases, the changes may simply be worsening of an old problem. Nevertheless, if a new type of arthritis is present, plenty of innovative treatments are available for improvement.

Rheumatoid Arthritis and Osteoarthritis

Kate, a pediatric nurse at a nearby hospital, has had pain and stiffness in her hand and knees due to osteoarthritis since age forty. This active mother of three managed the pain and stiffness by following the Exercise Treatment, using moist heat applications twice daily, and taking nonsteroidal anti-inflammatory drugs (NSAIDs). As long as she stayed on the Pain-Free Program, Kate reported no stiffness and very little pain.

Then, around age forty-five, Kate started to notice joint swelling and pain in new places—her wrists, shoulders, ankles, and feet. The pain and inflammation became so intense that she had to get up two hours earlier each day so the stiffness could subside before going to work at the hospital. Around noon each day, Kate had to nap during her lunch hour because of pain and fatigue.

When Kate came to the clinic for an evaluation, tests showed that she now had rheumatoid arthritis, along with the osteoarthritis. This explained the change in course of her arthritis and the increase in pain and stiffness in newly affected joints. Because she had early X-ray changes of rheumatoid arthritis, Kate immediately started methotrexate. Within three months, her pain was reduced substantially (more than 90 percent), and she no longer had morning stiffness. Kate started to work a full day without napping, and she resumed her Exercise Treatment.

The treatment for rheumatoid arthritis can include a DMARD medication, such as methotrexate. But for those with osteoarthritis alone, methotrexate gives no benefit. Kate continues taking the NSAID for both rheumatoid arthritis and osteoarthritis. This woman's experience shows that when arthritis symptoms change, it's wise to check with your rheumatologist to see if other treatments are available. Because Kate acted quickly and started the proper medications for rheumatoid arthritis, she was able to prevent destructive joint changes.

Fibromyalgia and Rheumatoid Arthritis

After experiencing constant pain, muscle tenderness, and fatigue for more than three years, thirty-seven-year-old Paula, a middle school music teacher, was finally given a diagnosis—fibromyalgia. Once she began the Exercise Treatment, twice-daily moist heat, and medications, including a COX-2 NSAID, imipramine, and an occasional non-narcotic pain medication, Paula began to notice a great improvement and was able to enjoy regular activities with family and friends.

Then one day some new symptoms emerged. Paula started noticing unusual swelling in her hands, wrists, feet, and ankles. She said that walking from her car to the school became extremely painful, and opening jars caused her great pain. She felt that she'd lost strength in her hands and was concerned because she taught piano lessons to children at school.

During the evaluation at our clinic, Paula's blood tests were positive for rheumatoid factor, and she had a very high sedimentation rate, a sign of inflammation. She started treatment for rheumatoid arthritis with methotrexate, which gave some relief, but she still had pain, swelling, stiffness, and fatigue. Paula then added Enbrel injections (see page 178). Within six weeks, she had noticed a dramatic improvement in joint pain and fatigue. Her activities have improved and she now has resumed her Exercise Treatment.

Temporomandibular Joint Syndrome (TMJ) and Rheumatoid Arthritis

Keith, a forty-three-year-old computer sales associate, has had rheumatoid arthritis for almost a decade. While his rheumatoid pain is well controlled using the Pain-Free Program, a few months ago, he began to notice new signs that were typical of TMJ. "I first noticed a problem with my left jaw while sitting in a sales meeting. My jaw felt weak, tired, and painful. Then it started to feel stiff in the mornings, which made it hard to open my mouth or even eat breakfast. As the day went on, I had a hard time talking and chewing. Within a few months, my right jaw was painful as well.

"As the jaw pain increased over a few weeks, I started to notice swelling. The area of pain spread up to my temples and down toward the lower part of my face. I could hear clicking in my jaws, and my ears felt stuffy with a popping sound at times."

After an evaluation, Keith was diagnosed with temporomandibular joint syndrome, which could have been made worse by recent job stress combined with some family problems. To ease the symptoms, I recommended that he use moist heat applications twice daily. Keith used a damp cloth that he heated in the microwave and then placed on the side of his jaw. He also used a warm shower on his jaws when the pain was intense. Keith said that while exercising his jaw, opening it as far as it could, he used ice cubes in a plastic bag to ease the pain and swelling.

Keith's dentist made a special mouthpiece for him to wear at night, and he also slept on a soft pillow while sleeping on his side. When the jaw was unusually painful, I suggested that Keith modify his diet and eat softer foods and avoid chewy or hard candy. Along with continued treatment for the rheumatoid arthritis, Keith's TMJ pain is now controlled and livable.

Osteoarthritis in the Knee and Injury

John had lived with osteoarthritis in his right knee with pain and stiffness for years since an injury he got in the service. When he retired from the army after twenty years, John remained active and continued exercise, and worked as a salesman with long hours of standing and walking. For about six months he noticed more swelling and pain than usual in the right knee and began to limit his activity. He had an injection of cortisone medication in the knee, which helped for a few days, but then the pain was worse than before.

When I saw John, his knee was swollen, and he had limited movement. X rays showed osteoarthritis and a fluid sample from the knee showed changes typical of this wear-and-tear type of arthritis. Magnetic resonance imaging (MRI) of John's knee showed that he had a damaged meniscus (cartilage) and a damaged anterior cruciate ligament. After referring John to an orthopedist for evaluation, he had successful arthroscopic surgery, and his knee pain lessened. After six weeks of rehabilitation, John resumed his usual exercise program, and the osteoarthritic knee pain returned to its previous manageable level.

Talk to Your Doctor about Your Pain

If you are still suffering with pain without any improvement after doing the Pain-Free Program for about four weeks, I encourage you to visit your doctor and see if there might be other causes of pain. Getting an early and accurate diagnosis, along with the proper treatment, can help you to feel pain-free so you can begin to enjoy your life again.

Arthritis and Pregnancy

When Jenny and her husband, Mike, decided to start a family, the first thing they did was come in together for a consultation. Thirty-one-year-old Jenny has had rheumatoid arthritis since her mid-twenties, and though her symptoms were well managed at this time, she had many questions about using medications during pregnancy, especially the toxic effect on the unborn fetus.

For women with arthritis who decide to start a family, it's important to plan for the care of both you and the baby. As you keep lines of communication open between your obstetrician and your doctor, you can be sure of the best ultimate outcome: a healthy baby *and* control of your arthritis.

Rheumatoid arthritis (RA) and systemic lupus erythematosus (SLE) are the most common types of arthritis in women of childbearing age. Moreover, the overall approach and treatment for the different types of arthritis during pregnancy are similar.

With both RA and SLE, the activity of the arthritis and the overall pregnancy outcome are affected by the timing of conception. For example, my patient Dana, a thirty-one-year-old, previously energetic woman, had finally begun to gain control over her debilitating joint pain, stiffness in the morning, and swollen hands resulting from RA. Now Dana is considering returning to work and wants to start her family.

Dana and I had a long discussion about timing conception, if possible, during the period of "quiet" activity of her RA, which means the pain and stiffness are fairly well controlled. I explained to Dana that the goal of controlling her arthritis during a pregnancy would be a delicate balance of maintaining pain-free quality of life for her RA with no adverse fetal outcome. Because methotrexate may cause damage to the growth of a fetus in several different organ systems, I suggested that she safely stop methotrexate at least three months before conception. Dana agreed to follow this plan and upon conception, she will continue to check in periodically.

Normal Changes with Pregnancy
In healthy women, pregnancy is often associated with anemia or low blood cell counts, rashes, joint pain, and even fatigue. For women with RA or SLE, these signs are often overwhelming and debilitating, as many suffer with these changes already. Thus, the goals for prenatal care in this situation include the following:

1. Control the underlying disease for the mother.
2. Minimize exposure of its treatment to the fetus.
3. Maximize nutrition.

Rheumatoid Arthritis
Most pregnant women with RA experience a significant improvement in their arthritis symptoms and usually have a favorable outcome. Studies show that starting in the first trimester of pregnancy, more than 75 percent of women with RA go into remission. It may be that the hormonal changes with pregnancy increase the production of an anti-inflammatory effect. For many women, this remission is an opportunity to have a trial off medications, or at least decreased doses of the medications that could have been potentially toxic to the fetus. About 90 percent of women with RA develop an exacerbation or worsening after the pregnancy, but then treatment that is more effective can be resumed after breast-feeding is finished.

Before delivery, your obstetrician and rheumatologist should make a careful evaluation of the extent and severity of the arthritic joints involved. For instance, vaginal delivery may be difficult for a woman with severe hip disease. If rheumatoid arthritis affects the cervical spine, your doctor can diagnose it by examining the neck and looking at X rays. This early evaluation will allow planning ahead of time to be sure of safe positioning and care of the cervical spine during labor and delivery.

Systemic Lupus Erythematosus

It is common for women with lupus to experience more flare-ups during their pregnancy. The flare-ups appear to occur before and within about six weeks after the actual delivery.

To minimize maternal and fetal risk and reduce the risk of flare-up during pregnancy, women with lupus should aim for remission or controlled lupus activity for at least six months before conception. If conception occurs during active symptoms, there is more than a 50 percent chance the disease will worsen throughout the pregnancy. Most increases in lupus activity are only mild, and less than 10 percent of patients develop a severe flare. If the woman has known kidney disease from the lupus before pregnancy, there is a risk of worsening with a pregnancy.

Fortunately, most flare-ups of lupus activity in pregnancy will quickly respond to increased doses of prednisone. If higher doses of prednisone are required to control the disease activity, your doctor will carefully monitor your blood pressure and blood sugar. A pregnant woman with lupus is at increased risk for developing high blood pressure, gestational (pregnancy-related) diabetes, urinary tract infections, and even pre-eclampsia, which usually occurs late in pregnancy with increased blood pressure, swelling of the hands and feet, and protein in the urine.

Arthritis Medications and Pregnancy

Obviously, the best situation during pregnancy is to avoid any medications that might have adverse effects on the mother or developing fetus. However, in women with rheumatic disease, the goal is to weigh the risks and benefits. Medication is necessary in most cases to keep the disease managed, so the goal becomes finding the safest and most effective treatment methods during this delicate time. Here are some of the medications your doctor may discuss during your preconception visit:

- *Aspirin.* Aspirin is not routinely recommended during pregnancy.
- *Nonsteroidal Anti-inflammatory Drugs (NSAIDs).* As discussed in Step 7, these medications are commonly used for most types of arthritis. It is not recommended to take NSAIDs during pregnancy.

- *Corticosteroids.* Corticosteroids are the first-line therapy in pregnancy for most flare-ups of any rheumatic disease, including RA and SLE. Your doctor can modify this treatment to include the safest form, such as injecting the medication directly into the painful joint if only a limited number of joints are involved. If the flare-up is more widespread, oral prednisone is still relatively safe with close monitoring for increased blood pressure, increased blood sugar, and more fluid retention causing uncomfortable swelling.

Children and Arthritis

Juvenile chronic arthritis (JCA), also known as juvenile idiopathic arthritis (JIA), is the most common childhood arthritis. An older name for it is juvenile rheumatoid arthritis (JRA). This disease may afflict up to 280,000 children in North America. We know that juvenile chronic arthritis has no relationship to adult onset rheumatoid arthritis for most children; thus the term *rheumatoid* was removed.

Types of Childhood Arthritis
There are three basic types of JIA based on associated symptoms and the number of joints involved from the first time the pain or symptoms are noticed.

1. Pauciarticular onset JIA: This includes those with less than five joints involved after the first six months of illness. This is the most common type, accounting for about half of all cases.
2. Polyarticular onset JIA: This is defined by having five or more joints involved after six months of the illness and is responsible for 30 to 40 percent of cases of JIA.
3. Systemic onset JIA, formerly called Still's disease: Affects children under sixteen years of age with intermittent high fevers and a rash. Any number of joints can be involved. This accounts for only 10 to15 percent of all cases of JIA.

A separate type of arthritis from JIA that can happen in childhood or teenage years is a group called the spondyloarthropathies. These have a tendency to involve the back and large joints in the legs, classically occurring in an adolescent male with low back pain or a swollen knee. Achilles tendonitis is also associated with this type of arthritis, and often all of these findings are attributed to a sports-related injury and the diagnosis is frequently delayed. Fortunately, spondyloarthropathy commonly responds well to NSAIDs and is not usually deforming.

Systemic onset JIA describes children less than sixteen years old who have intermittent high, spiking fevers, rash, and arthritis. They often appear quite ill and initially the doctor might think they have an infection that does not respond to antibiotics. Systemic JIA affects boys and girls equally at any age less than sixteen. Any number of joints can be involved, including the hips. The children are uncomfortable with swollen joints, but rarely actually cry out from pain. A child who appears well after six months will probably have a good prognosis. One-third of children with systemic JIA will remain ill for a long time.

Pain Assessment and Management in Children

Most children with arthritis will experience pain, stiffness, and even disability in different ways than adults. The intensity of the pain does not always correlate to the degree of the arthritis. In fact, children typically report less pain than adults do for fear of procedures (painful injections) or in efforts to please others. They may also imitate a parent's own response to pain.

Treatment

The goals of managing childhood arthritis are similar to adult arthritis, with control of pain and preventing disability most important. The medications selected for pain relief in adults are also chosen for children in appropriate doses for the size of the child.

First medications are usually nonsteroidal anti-inflammatory agents. NSAIDs reduce the number of swollen joints and decrease stiffness in the morning. Sometimes, if the pain is limited to one joint, an intra-articular injection is used. This is a relatively safe and effective early option.

If there is no improvement, your doctor may consider more aggressive medications for the underlying arthritis process itself, such as the disease-modifying anti-rheumatic agents (DMARDs), discussed on page 175. Typical traditional DMARDs include methotrexate, sulfasalazine, and plaquenil.

One of the biologic DMARDs or the newer TNF-blocking agents, such as etanercept (Enbrel), may also be used in children. Enbrel is used in the treatment of polyarticular onset JIA, although its role has yet to be specifically established.

Arthritis and Surgery

When you cannot manage your arthritis with conservative medical treatments and lifestyle changes, or if your daily activities are limited, you may want to talk with your doctor about surgical procedures. Surgery may help you become active again, including exercise. After surgery, a majority of patients enjoy much less pain and much improved mobility and activity. Of course, you must still continue the Pain-Free Program after surgery to get optimal benefit. The most common surgical options follow.

Total Joint Replacement

This procedure is most commonly performed on a knee or hip joint. Sometimes total joint replacement is performed on the shoulder and less frequently the elbow. Insertion of a prosthetic joint after removal of the previously damaged joint helps to relieve pain and increases function in those with osteoarthritis and rheumatoid arthritis if other treatments are not successful. Ironically, some new studies confirm that women with osteoarthritis who need total joint replacement may be less frequently offered the option to have the procedure done. Be advised: do not let gender be an issue as you seek to live pain-free!

Total joint replacement is most successful when performed before the development of a deformity (or before the joint becomes unstable or the muscles are too weak). Maximum pain relief is usually seen after twelve months, and then this relief may last for ten to fifteen years after total joint replacement. Problems associated with total joint replacement include loosening of the new joint, infection, and stiffness after the surgery. Today's advances in prosthetic joints and techniques give a successful outcome in 95 percent of hip and knee replacements in most centers.

Partial Knee Replacement (Unicompartmental Knee Arthroplasty)

In osteoarthritis, one alternative to replacing the entire knee joint (total knee arthroplasty) is to replace only one part (one compartment). This can be done in carefully selected patients when one side of the knee is more involved than the other. The medial (inside part of the knee) partial knee replacement has overall good results in pain relief and long-term satisfaction. However, this surgery is actually the best option for a minority of people with osteoarthritis of the knee. Partial knee arthroplasty is considered in younger people, with a higher rate of failure in heavy, physically active males. But most evidence shows more initial success, longevity, and fewer early complications than an osteotomy (see page 239).

Unfortunately, when trying to avoid replacing the whole knee with this surgery, there is the risk of needing a second surgery in the future if pain worsens. In that case, you then would have two separate surgeries and the potential for complications with each one. It is a difficult decision, one to make with the help of your orthopedic surgeon, especially if you have other medical problems. The important idea is to understand that there may be more than one alternative to total knee replacement when there is severe pain in your knee from your osteoarthritis.

Joint Irrigation (Lavage and/or Debridement)

This procedure is most commonly used in osteoarthritis. With a few small incisions the surgeon inserts an arthroscope with a camera on the tip into the arthritic joint. The contents of the joint are easily seen and the surgeon can smooth cartilage surfaces, remove pieces of broken cartilage, and repair ligaments. The presumed effect is to decrease pain by removing any irritating burden on the joint tissue. The benefit has been questioned for this procedure in knee osteoarthritis. Arthroscopic knee surgeries are the most frequently performed orthopedic procedure for arthritis.

Synovectomy

Synovectomy is more commonly performed in rheumatoid arthritis and is done early in a patient with only one joint involved and no X-ray changes of destruction. With this procedure, the surgeon will remove the inflamed synovium or joint lining. Synovectomy can be done as an open procedure or by arthroscopy. In general, arthroscopic procedures are associated with fewer complications and faster recovery than a more invasive, open surgical procedure. The relief in knee pain with synovectomy in rheumatoid arthritis may last up to five years.

Arthrodesis

This procedure involves surgical fusion of a severely damaged joint in which joint replacement is not recommended. The surgeon will permanently fix the joint, which relieves joint pain in rheumatoid or other inflammatory arthritis. Arthrodesis is most commonly performed on the wrist or ankle, joints in which total joint replacements have been less successful so far.

Osteotomy

For some patients with osteoarthritis in the knee who are very active, removal of a small wedge of bone from the knee can straighten the knee deformity in osteoarthritis and give excellent pain relief. This can be done in patients under age fifty before total joint replacement, as it allows full physical activity. The relief may last up to five to ten years, and this procedure can still be followed by total joint replacement.

Preoperative Considerations

If you are planning a procedure, you need to make regularly scheduled re-evaluations with your team of doctors before the operation and after it is completed. All professionals involved can participate in a quality discussion clearly defining the expectations for the surgery. Be sure you understand both the risks and benefits, location of incisions, usage of rods, drains, and prosthetic implants before having the surgery.

Talk openly with your team of doctors and ask what the postoperative period will entail. Make sure you are fully aware of the nature and duration of immobilization, use of casts or splints, and the schedule for any necessary physical therapy. For example, in many procedures, such as surgery on the hand, the post-op rehab period may help determine the best overall results. Be sure you understand what activities you will be able to do after full recovery.

Before surgery, you will probably undergo pre-op screening tests, including the following:

1. Basic blood work, including blood counts, kidney function, and blood glucose
2. Electrocardiogram (ECG)
3. Chest X ray
4. Urine analysis
5. Pregnancy test (if female)

Other tests will be determined by your doctor, depending on any coexisting medical problems, medications, your age, and the type and urgency of the surgery.

Special Considerations: Rheumatoid Arthritis

Some of the rheumatic diseases specifically present unique risks. The cornerstone of treatment of rheumatoid arthritis is early aggressive medical therapy. However, in some cases for prevention of future damage, or if there are permanent changes, surgery can improve the quality of life by giving pain relief and increased ability to function with daily tasks.

The goals of surgical procedures:

1. Reduce pain.
2. Increase function.
3. Prevent destruction of joints as well as correcting deformity.

In the past, orthopedic procedures for patients with rheumatoid arthritis were withheld until disease activity was quiet. By this point, deformity was more severe, and bones and muscles were weaker, so the results were not as good. Now, it is advised to consider preventative surgery at an earlier time with careful medical care combined with surgery.

When there are many joints damaged because of the arthritis, your doctor will discuss the order of operations. In general, the order is usually the spine, foot, hip, knee, wrist, shoulder, thumb, and elbow. However, each person is different.

More than 30 to 40 percent of patients with long-standing rheumatoid arthritis have involvement of the cervical spine. It's important to recognize the disease in the upper neck before any surgery, particularly prior to any anesthesia. Wearing a soft neck collar can be a safe "red flag" for increasing overall awareness before your surgery, when avoiding further injury is critical.

Surgical Risks

Researchers have found that taking 20 milligrams daily of prednisone (a supplementation of your body's own stress hormones) for at least two to three weeks anytime within the twelve months before surgery presents a risk during surgery. It is important to notify your surgeon of this medication history before the procedure, so you can be given extra doses of cortisone medications through the veins during and for a few days after the surgery.

Most joint surgery has an increased risk of forming a blood clot in the legs for several weeks postoperatively. This may occur even with no signs or symptoms. The concern is the clot traveling through the veins to the lungs, where there is an increased risk of death. Your surgeons are fully aware of this risk and are trained to give appropriate treatment with medications or methods such as devices that squeeze the legs or tight-fitting stockings.

While some patients have a previous history of heart disease, others with rheumatic diseases may have "silent" heart disease, which has not surfaced because of the severely limited activity level. Your doctor will decide if any further tests are needed before surgery.

Elderly

Older patients who require surgery face an increased risk of complications. Older patients have a unique and often more sensitive effect from anesthesia and other medications. There is also a higher rate of post-operative confusion, which usually is temporary. Your doctor will guide you for any special needs.

Post-Op

The duration of bed rest after the procedure will depend on the type of surgery. In many situations, on the day of the surgery (or the day after) a physical therapist may come to start some level of activity. The weeks after surgery are important to be sure you regain strength and movement in the joint. It's usually hard work, but well worth the effort. Your physical therapist and surgeon will guide you.

Tests You May Need

Getting an accurate diagnosis for your type of arthritis is crucial to living pain-free. Your doctor will make an accurate diagnosis after doing the following:

- Taking your medical history, including symptoms and family history of arthritis
- Performing a thorough physical examination
- Using various laboratory tests and imaging tests

Laboratory Tests

Laboratory tests can help to confirm the diagnosis—or to rule out different diseases. These tests will vary, depending on your signs and symptoms. Once the type of arthritis is properly identified, your doctor can prescribe a treatment regimen that helps to reduce pain and stiffness and increases your mobility. The goal, usually achievable, is for you to be able to do the activities you wish with reasonable comfort, with minimal side effects from medications.

Screening Laboratory Tests

A full blood count (FBC) measures the hemoglobin, red cells, white cells, and platelets and can find many of the common blood disorders, such as anemia, which can cause fatigue and tiredness. Thyroid tests can show if the thyroid is overactive or underactive, since either condition can aggravate the signs and symptoms of many types of arthritis. A high level of uric acid in the blood may indicate the presence of gout. A blood test for Lyme disease might help diagnose this treatable cause of arthritis. Still, beware that a positive blood test may not always mean that Lyme disease is the cause of your arthritis.

Sedimentation Rate

The sedimentation rate (ESR) measures how fast red blood cells fall to the bottom of a test tube. When inflammation is present, the blood's proteins clump together and become heavier than normal. The sedimentation rate can be high in almost any type of inflammatory arthritis, but in osteoarthritis the ESR rate is usually normal.

Rheumatoid Factor

The blood test for rheumatoid factor measures an abnormal protein in the blood and is positive in 70 to 80 percent of patients with rheumatoid arthritis. This test alone is not diagnostic of rheumatoid arthritis, as it's not present in all cases of rheumatoid arthritis and may be positive in other types of arthritis or in healthy people. Your doctor will do further tests to confirm the clinical diagnosis.

Antinuclear Antibody (ANA)

The ANA blood test checks for an abnormal protein in the blood commonly found in those who have connective tissue diseases or other autoimmune disorders, such as lupus. In fact, more than 90 percent of lupus patients have a positive blood test for antinuclear antibody. The ANA can also be positive in rheumatoid arthritis, after certain viral infections, or after taking certain medications.

Arthrocentesis

Arthrocentesis (joint aspiration) is often done to check the synovial (joint) fluid. Most arthritis causes swelling in the joints, which is a result of excess fluid production or swelling of the joint lining. If a sample of the joint fluid is removed with a small needle under local anesthesia, this can be a quick, almost painless, and inexpensive way to quickly tell a great deal about the cause of the arthritis. Different types of arthritis cause different changes in joint fluid. Normally there is only a very small amount of joint fluid to be found, and it is usually a yellow, almost clear, and somewhat thick (viscous) fluid that drips slowly from a needle.

- Osteoarthritis—joint fluid is not usually cloudy, may appear fairly close to normal, but increased in amount.
- Rheumatoid arthritis—joint fluid is cloudy, much thinner, and may also be greater in volume than normal.
- Gout—joint fluid is cloudy with microscopic crystals in the fluid, which can be viewed on examination of the fluid under a microscope.
- Infectious arthritis—joint fluid is usually thick, cloudy, and tests positive for infection.

Imaging Tests

The following imaging tests are commonly used to assess the joints and help decide the type of arthritis.

X Ray

X ray is an imaging test that uses X-ray electromagnetic energy beams to produce an image on film. X rays may be taken of the affected joints because specific changes can help to make the diagnosis of arthritis.

- Osteoarthritis—X rays will show changes in the joints with narrowing of the cartilage space. Spurs or extra growth of bone called osteophytes can usually be seen. In osteoarthritis of the spine, X rays show narrowing of the cartilage discs between the vertebral bones and spurs along the spine.
- Bursitis and tendonitis—minor changes may be apparent on X ray, including calcium deposits around the painful joint. More commonly, X rays are normal.
- Fibromyalgia—no X-ray changes in the joints, though doctors may order X rays to be sure no other problems are present to cause pain.
- Rheumatoid arthritis and other inflammatory arthritis—X rays show the earliest changes in the joints, which appear as tiny erosions at the edges of the bones of the hands, wrists, and feet. The erosions are a "red flag" indicating that a more serious form of rheumatoid arthritis might be brewing, one that can cause deformity and crippling as it progresses. This signals the need for early and aggressive treatment with effective medications to prevent long-term damage and deformity. The available medications can slow down or stop the progress of the arthritis in the bones, and it can be done before there are any outward or visible signs that severe arthritis is hiding.

- Ankylosing spondylitis—X rays show calcium bridges that form between the bones of the spine and abnormal sacroiliac joints.

Magnetic Resonance Imaging (MRI)

MRI uses magnetism, radio waves, and a computer instead of radiation to gather accurate information about internal organs and tissues. This imaging technique is often used to evaluate the knee, shoulder, spine, or other areas and can show abnormalities of cartilage and ligaments that routine X rays cannot show.

For patients with severe back pain, MRI can reveal the cause. It can show osteoarthritis and other types of arthritis in the spine and will show a ruptured disc, common in osteoarthritis patients, with more than 95 percent accuracy. MRI can also show lumbar stenosis, which is narrowing of the spinal canal that contains nerve roots coming from the spinal cord. Once the diagnosis is made, there can be effective treatment with medications or surgery.

MRI can be used at times for early detection of damage to joints in rheumatoid arthritis. So far, it is not used routinely because of the expense.

Some persons have feelings of claustrophobia because of the close situation in standard MRI equipment. Ask your doctor about the open MRI machine, which is less confining.

Computed Tomographic Scan (CT Scan)

A CT scan is a special X-ray procedure in which the X-ray beam moves around the body, taking pictures from various angles. This imaging technique is used to give a more detailed diagnosis of the internal organs and is especially useful for imaging bones in cases of severe back pain caused by arthritis. The CT scan can detect a ruptured disc in more than 85 percent of cases in the lumbar spine and can occasionally suggest an abnormality when the disc is actually normal. CT is more accurate than X ray to find infection, fracture of a bone, or cancer. With an acceptable level of radiation exposure, CT is done as an outpatient and may be less confining than MRI for those who might feel claustrophobic.

Bone Scan

A bone scan is used mainly when your doctor may suspect something more than arthritis, such as an infection, cancer, or fracture of a bone. It can detect abnormal areas of bone produced by these problems in all parts of the body's skeleton. The test is painless except for the injection of a small amount of radioactive dye followed in a few hours by a scan of the body while the patient lies on an X-ray table.

Myelogram

The myelogram requires an injection of dye into the spinal canal (a procedure similar to a spinal tap) through a needle to show the rupture of a disc or other problems. Normally the dye would fill the spinal canal as well as the nerve root sheaths, giving a revealing outline for an X ray. Yet, in an abnormal myelogram, there is an absence of dye in a specific area. This is called a "filling defect" and indicates that the nerve root or spinal cord is pinched or compressed. This test detects the ruptured disc.

The myelogram has more discomfort, is more invasive, requires an injection, and has a greater possibility of an unwanted side effect such as a headache. Some experts now recommend MRI of the lumbar spine; then, if there is not a clear answer, a myelogram is performed. A CT scan may be combined with myelogram to improve the accuracy of diagnosis, especially if a small piece of disc has broken off and is pressing on a nerve away from its root between the vertebrae.

Electromyelogram (EMG) and Nerve Conduction Study

These two tests are used in combination to diagnose sources of pain, including carpal tunnel syndrome and other nerve or muscle disorders. An electromyelogram measures the activity of the muscles supplied by the nerves that are being irritated by your ruptured or herniated disc. A nerve conduction study tests the velocity in which the nerve transmits its signal. In other words, if the nerve is pinched, its ability to transmit a signal is reduced. Abnormal muscle activity and slowed nerve conduction may suggest a pinched or irritated nerve from a disc rupture.

Arthrogram

In this test, dye is injected into a joint to show the structures in detail. It can be painful and is not used very often since MRI may give similar information without as much discomfort.

Types of Arthritis

Ankylosing Spondylitis

This type of arthritis is caused by inflammation of the joints of the lower back (the lumbar spine and sacroiliac joints), which causes back pain. Ankylosing spondylitis is more common in men and usually begins in the lower back but can cause a gradual limitation of motion in the entire spine, including the neck. Back and neck exercises (see page 263) are especially important to help keep normal motion and posture in the back and neck.

Symptoms: Lower back pain; morning stiffness; fatigue; pain in hips, shoulders, or other joints.

Diagnosis: Patient history and symptom discussion; physical examination; X-ray evidence; positive blood test for HLA-B27 antigen (inherited factor).

Treatment: Twice-daily moist heat applications; back and neck exercises; NSAIDs; your doctor can advise further medication and other steps if you do not have good control of pain, stiffness, and/or function.

Bursitis and Tendonitis

In bursitis pain is caused by inflammation of the sac that lubricates tendons as they move through their sheath. There is pain on movement at the shoulder or other areas. This is commonly caused by overuse or wear and tear.

In tendonitis, pain is usually most severe at the point that the tendon attaches to the bone, such as at the elbow, in tennis elbow or golfer's elbow. This also is usually from overuse or wear and tear.

Symptoms: Pain in the affected bursa or tendon, with pain that may be severe on movement of the shoulder (bursitis or tendonitis); squeezing handgrip as in tennis or golf can cause pain at the elbow (tendonitis).

Diagnosis: Made on clinical examination, usually with severe pain in a localized area around the shoulder, elbow, or other affected joint. X rays can show that other more serious problems are not causing the pain.

Treatment: For bursitis, moist heat and rest; NSAID treatment for 1–2 weeks; local injection if not improved; gradual increase in exercise with your physical therapist. For tendonitis, moist heat and rest; NSAID treatment for 1–2 weeks; and local injection or orthopedic surgery option if not improved.

Carpal Tunnel Syndrome

This common problem is caused by pressure on the median nerve in the wrist, which supplies part of the palm of the hand, the thumb, and adjacent fingers. Carpal tunnel syndrome (CTS) can result from many types of arthritis, from repetitive use or injury, and many other causes.

Symptoms: Numbness, tingling, and a "pins-and-needles" sensation in the thumb and adjacent fingers. Symptoms are more common at night or when you drive a car and are usually relieved when you move or reposition the affected wrist.

Diagnosis: Patient history and description of symptoms, physical examination, nerve conduction tests.

Treatment: Twice daily applications of moist heat; wrist exercises; wrist splints; NSAIDs; local injection; surgery.

Childhood Arthritis (Juvenile Chronic Arthritis, Juvenile Rheumatoid Arthritis)

Arthritis in children occurs before age sixteen and can have several forms with many of the same findings as adult rheumatoid arthritis. The outlook for improvement is better in children as 50 percent or more of the cases usually improve, and in many cases, the arthritis disappears altogether.

Symptoms: (see Adult Rheumatoid Arthritis). Joint pain and swelling can attack only one joint, such as a knee, or many joints. Some cases have fever and little apparent joint swelling.

Diagnosis: Patient history and description of symptoms; physical examination; X rays; and blood tests.

Treatment: This is similar to adult rheumatoid arthritis but must be individualized for each child. Talk to your pediatrician or pediatric rheumatologist.

Chronic Back Pain

Back pain affects half of all Americans annually. In most cases, the cause of the pain is in the muscles, tendons, and other soft tissues of the back and neck or by osteoarthritis in the spine. When the pain lasts more than a few weeks, the specific causes of this chronic pain should be found and addressed so treatment can be planned. Other medical problems such as kidney stones, ruptured discs, aneurysm of the aorta, or cancer can also cause back pain. Each of these causes has different and effective treatments available.

Symptoms: If your back pain includes the following warning signs, talk to your doctor for a proper diagnosis:

- Pain that awakens you from sleep
- Pain that worsens when you cough or sneeze
- Pain that travels down one or both legs
- Difficulty passing or controlling bowels or urination.

Diagnosis: Patient history and description of symptoms; physical examination; X rays; and blood tests. It may be necessary to have an MRI (magnetic resonance imaging), which can detect pressure on nerves as they exit the spine, or CT scan (computerized tomography), which can also be used to detect abnormalities in the nerves and discs of the lower back.

Treatment: Twice-daily moist heat applications; gentle exercises; and NSAIDs. If you do not find relief in two weeks, check with your doctor for further ways to control chronic back pain.

Fibromyalgia

Fibromyalgia is diagnosed when there is chronic widespread pain throughout the back and other areas along with typical tender trigger points as long as there is not another cause to explain the symptoms.

Symptoms: Severe, widespread pain; specific tender points over the body; severe fatigue with no other medical cause apparent; difficulty sleeping; irritable bowel syndrome; difficulty concentrating ("fibro fog"); headaches. Depression is common.

Diagnosis: Patient history and description of symptoms; physical examination; check for widespread pain and trigger points. Laboratory tests are normal in fibromyalgia.

Treatment: Twice-daily moist heat applications (see page 14); exercises on page 263; medications listed on page 155.

Gout

Gout is caused by a high level of uric acid in the blood, which results in deposits of sodium urate crystals around the joints and sometimes in the kidneys as stones. If left untreated, the attacks become more frequent and severe damage to cartilage may affect the performance of the joint.

Symptoms: Severe pain and swelling commonly in the large toe or foot, which can last for weeks. Sometimes an acute gouty arthritis attack has a sudden onset at nighttime. The pain can be so severe that the weight of the sheets causes pain in the foot.

Diagnosis: Patient history and description of symptoms; physical examination of the affected joints; blood test showing high uric acid. To seal the diagnosis, your doctor may remove a sample of joint fluid to examine for uric acid crystals.

Treatment: While untreated attacks may last up to weeks at a time, gouty arthritis is easily treated with nonsteroidal anti-inflammatory drugs (NSAIDs), including Celebrex, Vioxx, Mobic, Bextra, Indocid, Voltarol or Didofenac. Colchicine is an old drug that can still be very effective. After the attack is over, medications including allopurinol can prevent future attacks by lowering the level of uric acid in the blood.

Infectious Arthritis

When bacterial or other infections attack the joints, they sometimes cause arthritis. This might happen following an infection in the skin around the joint or when bacteria travel from another part of the body to the joint. In most cases, just one joint, such as the knee, is involved at a time. People who have diabetes mellitus, sickle cell anemia, HIV infection, or are IV drug users are at highest risk.

Lyme disease is one type of infection that can cause arthritis. It is caused by the bite of a tick infected with the Lyme disease organism (*Borrelia burgdorferi*). The first stage after the bite presents flulike symptoms with or without a rash around the tick bite. About 10 percent of Lyme disease cases progress, with some people developing symptoms such as headache, nerve involvement, or even heart disease. Some people continue on to the third stage, which causes chronic arthritis with pain and swelling in the joints that can mimic rheumatoid arthritis.

Symptoms: For infectious arthritis, pain in the affected joint with swelling, warmth, redness, and commonly fever. For Lyme arthritis, in early stages, you might have flulike symptoms, rash; in later stages, you might have headache, nerve or heart involvement, joint pain and swelling.

Diagnosis: For infectious arthritis, patient history and description of symptoms, physical examination of the affected joints, blood tests, and analyzing a sample of the joint fluid to determine which type of infection is present. The joint fluid is removed using a syringe or sometimes by an operation.

Treatment: Antibiotics are most effective for infectious arthritis since they work to kill the organism that causes the problem. Surgery may be used for treatment to better remove all of the infection.

Lyme Disease (see Infectious Arthritis)

Osteoarthritis (OA)

This common type of arthritis is known as the "wear and tear" type and usually affects people over age fifty or those who have an injured joint, such as an athletic injury of the knee. The cartilage, which usually cushions the joint, becomes worn and less efficient. Osteoarthritis is most common in the joints that bear the weight of the body—the knees, hips, and spine, and in joints that have been injured. OA usually comes on gradually over the years and is more common in those who are over-weight.

Symptoms: Occasional pain and stiffness with increasing pain and swelling in the joint over time; prominent swelling from joint fluid or enlargement of the bone around the joint by bone spurs; pain is most noticeable when using the particular joint.

One form of OA that is less known affects the hands of younger women in their thirties or forties. This type of arthritis may be inherited and causes pain and swelling, with enlargement of the finger joints, but does not usually cause severe arthritis in other joints.

Diagnosis: Patient history and description of symptoms, and physical examination of the affected joints. X rays can show bone spurs and the narrowing of joint cartilage in osteoarthritis but not the destructive process that happens with rheumatoid arthritis (see page 257).

Treatment: Moist heat and exercises for the joints affected, as on pages 14 and 263. Over-the-counter acetaminophen, ibuprofen, or naprox-en might control your pain. Glucosamine may also be added to give relief and might delay the progress of the cartilage loss. If these don't help enough, find the most effective NSAID for you; page 166 lists the COX-2 NSAIDs, which are safer if you must take an NSAID on a regular basis. For the knee, injections of hyaluronic acid medications may give relief for months. After years, surgery may be needed to keep you pain-free and active.

Polymyalgia Rheumatica and Temporal Arteritis

This type of arthritis causes severe pain and stiffness in the shoulders, upper arms, hips, and thighs. Polymyalgia rheumatica causes pain and stiffness of the muscles and tissues around the joints.

Symptoms: Often, sudden onset of pain and stiffness, difficulty sleeping; severe stiffness on awakening in the morning; fever; and weight loss. Some people with polymyalgia develop severe headaches, jaw pain, and changes in vision. This happens when temporal arteritis (page 260) is present. A fast diagnosis is crucial to prevent loss of vision and other complications.

Diagnosis: Patient history and description of symptoms; physical examination of the affected joints; and blood tests. The sedimentation rate, the most important lab test, is almost always abnormally elevated in polymyalgia rheumatica and in temporal arteritis. A simple biopsy (removal of a tissue sample for examination under a microscope) of a temporal artery at the side of the head can help to confirm the diagnosis.

Treatment: Low doses of prednisone. If temporal arteritis is present, higher doses of prednisone can control the disease and pain should diminish in a few days, and the prednisone is continued for a number of months, then gradually lowered. Treatment may last a few months to two years.

Pseudogout

This arthritis mimics gout because it causes pain and swelling in a joint, similar to an attack of gouty arthritis. Pseudogout can affect the wrist, knee, or other joints and can last for weeks.

Symptoms: Sudden onset of pain and swelling in affected joint(s).

Diagnosis: Patient history and description of symptoms; physical examination of the affected joints; X rays that show calcification in the cartilage near the joint; and analysis of joint fluid sample that shows the typical calcium pyrophosphate crystals—different from the uric acid crystal of gout.

Treatment: Nonsteroidal anti-inflammatory drugs (NSAIDs) and/or local injection of a cortisone medication.

Psoriatic Arthritis

Psoriasis is a skin disease that causes a red, scaly rash most commonly over the elbows, knees, hands, and other areas. About 10 percent of those with this disease also develop a form of arthritis that mimics rheumatoid arthritis and can cause permanent deformities and damage in the joints.

Symptoms: Pain and swelling in the hands, wrists, elbows, shoulders, knees, ankles, feet, and spine; morning stiffness; and fatigue similar to that of rheumatoid arthritis.

Diagnosis: The diagnosis is usually made when arthritis similar to rheumatoid arthritis is present in a patient with psoriasis and a negative rheumatoid factor blood test.

Treatment: Twice-daily moist heat applications; exercises (as described for rheumatoid arthritis on page 263); NSAIDs. If not enough improvement or if there are permanent changes on your X rays, then a second medication (usually methotrexate, Enbrel, Remicade, or another biologic DMARD) is added to help prevent long-term joint damage.

Raynaud's Phenomenon

This condition can happen in many different types of arthritis or it can affect otherwise healthy persons.

Symptoms: Fingers become pale or white when they are exposed to cold such as a freezer, refrigerator, or even holding a cold glass. The fingers usually turn blue or red within a few minutes as the blood circulation returns to normal.

Diagnosis: Patient history of cold and other triggers causing discoloration in the fingers. The doctor will make sure no other problems are causing the Raynaud's phenomenon.

Treatment: If the episodes cannot be controlled by avoiding the triggering situations (such as by wearing gloves for cold exposure), medications may help to control the symptoms.

Reactive Arthritis

The body's defense may respond to an infection with an inflammatory reaction that triggers arthritis. In these cases, the arthritis may cause joint pain and swelling, which looks very much like rheumatoid or other types of arthritis.

Symptoms: Pain and swelling in the hands, wrists, elbows, shoulders, knees, ankles, and feet. Often the symptoms are acute and may be self-limited to a few weeks or months.

Diagnosis: Diagnosis is made after discussion and examination and with the help of blood tests and X rays, since there is no single test that confirms this diagnosis.

Treatment: Chronic reactive arthritis is treated with medications similar to those used for rheumatoid arthritis (see page 258).

Reiter's Syndrome

This type of arthritis is most common in younger men. Those affected may also have urethritis (inflammation of the urethra), which causes painful urination and discharge from the penis, eye inflammation (conjunctivitis), or diarrhea. Reiter's syndrome may resolve after a few weeks and can return in cycles. Or, in some cases, it can become chronic along with the potential for joint damage. The treatment is similar to treatment for rheumatoid arthritis.

Repetitive Stress Injury

Repetitive stress injury refers to injury from repetitive use of the hand and wrist, such as working at a computer. In the wrist, the repeated use may result in inflammation around the median nerve, causing symptoms of carpal tunnel syndrome with "pins and needles" feelings or a numbness sensation in the thumb and fingers. Treatment involves correcting the work situation, if possible, to avoid the repetitive injury to the wrist. If symptoms persist, treatment includes local injection of the carpal tunnel, use of a splint to maintain proper position, or treatment with surgery.

Rheumatoid Arthritis (RA)

Rheumatoid arthritis is the most common of type of inflammatory arthritis and can affect almost any age. RA usually comes on gradually and causes pain and swelling in the hands, wrists, elbows, shoulders, knees, ankles, and feet. This serious form of arthritis can cause destruction and deformity in joints if uncontrolled. Newer medications are breakthroughs in control of pain and prevention of deformities.

Symptoms: Morning stiffness, joint pain, fatigue, and weight loss. Many patients find the fatigue to be as limiting as the joint pain, and fever may accompany this, too. The joint pain and swelling make it difficult to complete even routine daily tasks such as getting dressed, opening jars, writing, and working.

   With rheumatoid arthritis, the affected joints enlarge and can become deformed. Sometimes joints may freeze in one position (contractures), making movement difficult or impossible to extend or open. About 30 to 40 percent of those with rheumatoid arthritis have hard bumps (nodules) just under the skin, usually near the diseased joints.

Diagnosis: Patient history and description of symptoms, and physical examination of the affected joints. X rays of the joints may show small areas of erosion or destruction of the edges of the bones around the joints. Blood tests may show the presence of rheumatoid factor, a protein that is present in 70 to 80 percent of cases. The sedimentation rate is usually above normal.

Treatment: Twice-daily moist heat applications; exercises as outlined on page 29; NSAIDs. If you must take NSAIDs daily, consider the COX-2 NSAIDs, which are safer for long-term treatment. If the pain and stiffness are not controlled early in the disease, or if there are changes on X rays, the traditional and biologic DMARDs control the pain and stiffness and delay future joint damage. Methotrexate is most commonly used first, and then if there is not enough improvement, one of the biologic DMARDs (see list on page 177) is added.

Scleroderma

Scleroderma causes tightening of the skin of the fingers, as well as joint pain and stiffness. The disease usually begins gradually and may spread to involve large areas of the skin and face. Over time, the skin loses its flexibility and the fingertips may develop ulcers, which are difficult to heal. Scleroderma may affect internal organs, most commonly with heartburn, indigestion, esophageal disease, or lung disease. In severe cases, the lungs and kidneys may be affected, too.

Symptoms: The skin over the hands and fingers may change first. Raynaud's phenomenon is common with the fingers turning white with cold exposure (see page 256). The arthritis can affect the hands, wrists, elbows, shoulders, knees, ankles, feet, and jaw. Tightening skin may limit the use of the hands for daily tasks and may change facial appearance. Heartburn, indigestion, and shortness of breath may be problems.

Diagnosis: Patient history and description of symptoms, and physical examination to see the typical skin changes. Blood tests can help confirm the diagnosis in some early cases of scleroderma.

Treatment: There is no excellent treatment for this type of arthritis, but the focus is on maintaining good pain control, preventing the loss of joint use, and managing internal organ disease.

Sjogren's Syndrome

With Sjogren's syndrome, the glands that usually produce moisture fail to prevent dryness in the eyes, nose, and mouth. This is most common in patients who also have rheumatoid arthritis, but it can happen alone or with other types of arthritis.

Symptoms: Dryness of the eyes that affects vision and may damage the cornea; eye infections; mouth dryness; dental cavities; swollen glands on the side of the face (parotid glands).

Diagnosis: Patient history and description of symptoms, physical examination, and simple biopsy of the lip or other area.

Treatment: Artificial tears for the eyes; maintaining moisture in the mouth; seeing your dentist frequently to prevent further tooth decay. Medications, including Sialgen or Evoxac, are available to help improve moisture.

Systemic Lupus Erythematosus, SLE (Lupus)

In lupus the joints become inflamed with pain and swelling. But this type of arthritis also causes inflammation and damage in internal organs. Although the kidney is most commonly affected, lupus can attack the heart, brain, skin, and almost any organ. This internal organ disease can be life threatening, but is treatable if detected early. Lupus is more common in women, particularly African-American women. The cause is not known.

Symptoms: Almost any symptom can happen—pain and swelling in the hands, wrists, elbows, shoulders, knees, ankles, and feet; fatigue; fever; rash, especially rash across the face (butterfly rash); sun sensitivity;

Choosing the Best Doctor

If you need to see a specialist, try to select a health care professional who is best qualified to diagnose and treat arthritis. Some areas to consider include:

- The doctor is board certified in rheumatology (specialist in arthritis) or a related field.
- The doctor is trustworthy and has an excellent reputation in the community.
- The doctor is involved in academic pursuits, such as research, writing, or teaching.
- The doctor has hospital privileges at excellent hospitals near you.
- The doctor accepts your particular health insurance or is on the selected medical panel for your HMO.
- The doctor's staff is attentive, professional, and accessible for questions concerning your health or insurance/payment issues.

hair loss; chest pain; shortness of breath from heart or lung disease; kidney disease; blood clots; headache; seizures; and strokes.

Diagnosis: Over 90 percent of patients with SLE have a positive blood test for antinuclear antibody (ANA). Other blood tests can help confirm that SLE is the diagnosis. Your doctor will do a careful physical examination to find the extent of internal organ disease so treatment is most effective. You may see a specialist for one of the specific internal organ disorders.

Treatment: Cortisone-type medications at certain times, along with other medications, can control the disease. It is important to have close follow-up by your rheumatologist and other doctors to ensure the best possible outcome. The medications themselves can cause side effects, which may be minimized or avoided.

Temporal Arteritis

With temporal arteritis, you have inflammation in the arteries, including the temporal arteries, which can cause headache, loss of vision, and stroke, if untreated.

Symptoms: Most commonly, headache; severe or new jaw pain when chewing; visual changes; fever; fatigue; and weight loss. Polymyalgia rheumatica can occur along with temporal arteritis, causing severe pain and stiffness in the shoulders, arms, hips, and thighs.

What to Bring to Your Appointment

Bring the following to your doctor's visit:

- A list of health concerns, including signs and symptoms of arthritis
- A description of the pain, including location, intensity, and known triggers
- Past illnesses and medications
- A list of current medications
- Any natural dietary supplement you are taking (herbs, vitamins/ minerals, other)
- Family health history, including history of arthritis
- Information on previous surgeries
- Lifestyle habits, including diet, exercise, and smoking

Diagnosis: Patient history and examination. With temporal arteritis, there is almost always an abnormal sedimentation rate. A simple temporal artery biopsy under local anesthesia is the most accurate way to diagnose the disease.

Treatment: Prednisone, in higher doses than for polymyalgia, usually 40–60 mg daily, then gradually lowered over months as there is improvement.

Exercises

Use the following stretches daily, including before exercise or performing any physical task. You will find that stretching helps to ease stiffness and allows you to be more active throughout the day.

Chest and Mid-Back
Place a broom or a long pole behind your back and across your shoulders with your hands supporting the long handle or poke at each end. Then slowly rotate your torso to the left; repeat this movement in the opposite direction.

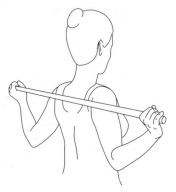

Figure A.1.

Chest and mid-back stretches.

Shoulders
Hold a broom handle or long pole with both hands over your head and slowly stretch from side to side like a pendulum several times. Then place

the handle or pole at shoulder level in front of you and gently turn to the right as far as it is comfortable, then to the left. Repeat several times.

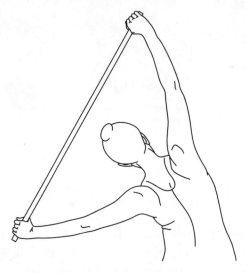

Figure A.2.

Shoulder stretches.

Neck

Place one hand on the side of your head just above the ear and gently push as if you are trying to place your ear to your shoulder. Gradually build pressure while allowing no movement to occur. Hold and then relax.

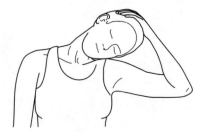

Figure A.3.

Neck stretches.

Legs and Hamstrings

Stand upright and put foot on bench (or step). Slowly bend forward at the hip while keeping your back straight. Alternate to the other leg and repeat exercise. You should feel the stretch behind your thigh.

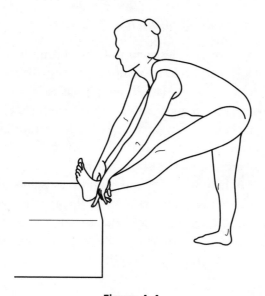

Figure A.4.

Leg and hamstring stretches.

Back

This exercise will help keep your posture straight and alleviate stress on the back and hips. Lie on your back with your knees bent and feet flat on the floor and hip-width apart. While contracting your abdominal muscles, press your lower back against the floor. You will feel your pelvis rock (tilt) toward your shoulders. The bottom of your buttocks and your pelvis will come slightly of the floor during the action.

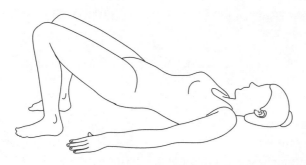

Figure A.5.

Back stretches.

Range-of-Motion Exercises

The following exercises are designed to build flexibility and strength in the neck, shoulders, and back. It is important to work toward a goal of doing these exercises twice a day, 20 repetitions each. At first, you may only be able to do 1 to 2 repetitions of each exercise. That is a reasonable start. However, as you gain strength and mobility, move into the twice-daily, 20 repetitions each routine. If you have any pain or unusual feeling, stop the exercise and contact your physician.

Sometimes it is helpful to get some gentle assistance from a family member or friend. Your physician or physical therapist can show you how.

A word of caution: Do not hold your breath while performing any exercise. If you feel pain with any of the suggested exercises, stop the exercise and discuss it with your physician.

Neck Range-of-Motion Exercises

It is important to build strength in the neck as well as improve the mobility and flexibility. Arthritis causes inflammation, pain, and stiffness, and these range-of-motion exercises will enable your body to perform more effectively. While flexion should be done standing, the rest of the neck exercises can be performed sitting or standing, whichever is more comfortable for you.

Flexion
While standing, look down and bend your chin forward to the chest. If you feel stiffness or pain, do not force the movement. Go as far as you can without straining yourself. If your arthritis pain worsens with this or any exercise, stop until you have talked to your physician or physical therapist.

Extension
Look up and bend your head back as far as possible without forcing any movement.

Lateral Flexion
Tilt your left ear to your left shoulder (but do not raise the shoulder). If you feel pain or resistance, do not force the motion.

Now tilt the ear to the right shoulder just as you did for the left ear (see figure A.6).

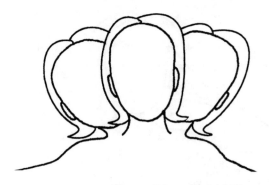

Figure A.6.

Lateral flexion.

Rotation

Turn to look over your left shoulder. Try to make your chin even with your shoulder. Go as far as is comfortable, but do not force the movement.

Now turn and look over your right shoulder, as you did with the left.

Neck Isometric Exercises

Neck isometric exercises are more advanced exercises to help strengthen the muscles of the neck. Gently and gradually try these after range of motion of your neck is improved as much as possible. Again, do not hold your breath.

Isometric Flexion

Place hand on your forehead. Try to look down while resisting the motion with your hand. Hold for 6 seconds. Count out loud.

Place your hands on the back of your head. Try to look up and back while resisting the motion with your hands. Hold for 6 seconds. Count out loud.

Isometric Lateral Flexion

Hold your head straight. Place your left hand just above your left ear. Try to tilt your head to the left but resist the motion with your left hand. Hold for 6 seconds. Count out loud.

Now place your right hand just above your right ear. Try to tilt your head to the right but resist the movement with your right hand. Hold for 6 seconds. Count out loud.

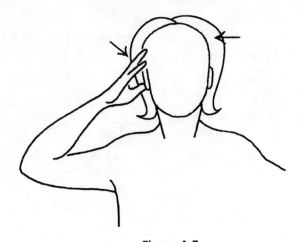

Figure A.7.

Isometric lateral flexion.

Isometric Rotation

Place your left hand above your ear and near your left forehead. Now try to look over your left shoulder, but resist the motion with your left hand. The hand should not be placed on the jaw. Hold for 6 seconds. Count out loud.

Now place your right hand above your ear and near your right forehead. Now try to look over your right shoulder, but resist the motion with your right hand. Hold for 6 seconds. Count out loud.

Shoulder Range-of-Motion Exercises

The following five range-of-motion exercises will increase the flexibility of the shoulders and arms. Increasing the number of exercises can increase the strength of the arms.

Shoulder External Rotation

This exercise increases the motion you use to comb your hair. You may sit, stand, or lie down to do these exercises.

Clasp your hands behind your head. Pull your elbows together until they are as close as possible in front of your chin. Separate the elbows to the side as much as possible.

Repeat this, gradually increasing to 5, then 10, then up to 20 repetitions. You may repeat these two or three times daily.

Shoulder Internal Rotation

Shoulder internal rotation increases the flexibility of the shoulders. Using the same motions women use to fasten a bra in the back or men use to put a wallet in a back pocket, move your arms in the position as shown in figure A.8. This exercise is best done standing and is often done in the shower using a washcloth to wash your upper back or a towel to dry it.

Put your hand behind your back. Then put the other hand behind your back and cross the wrist as shown in the picture. Return the hands to rest at your side.

Repeat this, gradually increasing to 5, then 10, then up to 20 repetitions. Repeat twice daily.

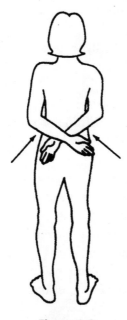

Figure A.8.

Shoulder internal rotation.

Shoulder Flexion

Shoulder flexion holds both arms down at your sides. Raise the left arm straight up and reach overhead toward the ceiling. Now do the same with the right arm. Continue this motion as you alternate left-right-left-right. Repeat this, gradually increasing to 5, then 10, then up to 20 repetitions, and repeat the exercise twice daily.

Shoulder Abduction

Raise both arms straight out away from your sides, then raise each arm overhead toward the ceiling and up above your head. Do this with your palm up or palm down.

If this exercise is painful while sitting or standing, you can also do it while lying on your bed. Use a stick (a broom handle will do) as you raise your arms, hold the stick with both hands and keep the arms straight, up over your head as far as possible. The strength of the less painful arm will help the painful arm move more easily.

Repeat this exercise, gradually increasing to 5, then 10, then 20 repetitions two or three times a day.

Once you have mastered the exercise, go to the second part. This involves raising your arms out to the side, one a time, then slowly make big circles.

Repeat this exercise, gradually increasing to 5, then 10, then 20 repetitions two or three times a day.

Shoulder Girdle Rotation

This exercise can be done in a sitting or standing position and is fun to do during the day to relieve neck and shoulder tension and maintain shoulder girdle flexibility.

Roll shoulders in a forward circle; raise shoulders toward the ears in a shrugging motion. Roll shoulders back and chest out as in a military stance. Lower the shoulders and bring the shoulders forward. Think of it as a simple shoulder roll in a circle. Now reverse the process, rolling your shoulder girdle in a backward circle.

Repeat this exercise, gradually increasing to 5, then 10, then 20 repetitions two or three times a day if possible.

Back Exercises

As you do the following strengthening exercises, it is important that you breathe properly while holding the position. Counting to 6 aloud will enable you to do this easily. If you experience shortness of breath, stop and talk to your doctor or physical therapist.

Cheek to Cheek

This is a convenient exercise because you can do it anywhere, anytime, and practically in any position. It strengthens the muscles of the buttocks that help support the back and the legs. When sitting, you will actually raise up out of the chair because of the contraction of the muscle groups in the buttocks.

Press your buttocks together and hold for a 6-second count. Relax and repeat. Gradually increase up to 5, then 10, then 20 repetitions.

Do this exercise frequently during the day.

Pelvic Tilt

This is one of the best exercises you can do to strengthen your abdominal muscles, which in turn help support your back. It will also help tone your stomach muscles. Do this exercise lying on your back in bed or on the floor, whichever is more comfortable.

Relax and raise your arms above your head. Keep your knees bent. Now comes the tricky part! Tighten the muscles of your lower abdomen and your buttocks at the same time to flatten your back against the floor or bed. Hold the flat-back position for a 6-second count. Now relax and repeat.

Repeat this exercise 2 or 3 times to start and work up gradually to 5, then 10, then 20 repetitions.

If you have trouble, contact your physical therapist or physician and have them demonstrate the exercise. This may be particularly necessary if you want to do this exercise standing up or sitting in a chair.

Bridging

This exercise strengthens the muscles in the back.

Lie on your back on the floor or in bed and bend (flex) your hips and knees. Now lift your hips and buttocks off the bed or floor 4 to 6 inches,

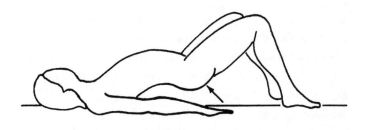

Figure A.9.

A bridging exercise.

forcing the small of the back out flat; tighten the buttock and hip muscles to maintain this position. Hold this position for a count of 6 seconds. Now, relax and lower your hips and buttocks to the floor or bed.

Repeat this exercise, gradually increasing up to 5, then 10, then 20 repetitions as tolerated. Repeat this twice daily if possible.

Partial Sit-Up

This is one of the more vigorous exercises. Its purpose is to build abdominal strength to give the back greater support.

To do this exercise lie on your back on the bed or on the floor, whichever is more comfortable, with your knees bent.

Raise your head and shoulder blades off the floor or bed. Hold that position for a 6-second count. Slowly return to the beginning position of lying on your back. Repeat.

Start this exercise slowly with 1 or 2 repetitions until your body adjusts. Gradually increase to 5, then 10 repetitions.

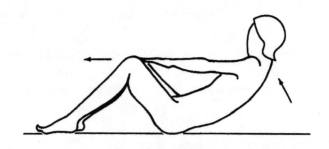

Figure A.10.

A partial sit-up exercise.

Back Extension

For this exercise to strengthen the back muscles, lie on your bed or on the floor in a prone (stomach-down) position. A pillow may be used under the stomach to help make this position more comfortable.

Raise your head, arms, and legs off the floor. Do not bend your knees. This must be done with your body straight in extension. Hold for 6 seconds while you count out loud. Relax and repeat.

Gradually increase up to 5, then 10 repetitions. If you experience discomfort, check with your physician or physical therapist before you continue.

Cat Camel

Do not do this exercise for strengthening the back muscles if you have very painful knees, ankles, or hands as it places pressure on these areas.

The position for this exercise is a crawling position. Hands must be directly under your shoulders. Take a deep breath and arch your back as a frightened cat does, lowering your head. Hold that position while you count the 6 seconds out loud. Now exhale and drop the arched back slowly, raising your head.

Start this exercise slowly with 1 or 2 repetitions. Increase up to 5 and then 10 repetitions if possible.

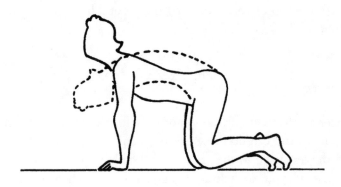

Figure A.11.

A cat-camel exercise.

Wall Push

This exercise is good for the back because it encourages the body extension positions.

Stand spread eagle with your back against a solid wall. Now arch your back inward slowly.

Gradually increase repetitions from 1 to 5 or more. This exercise is fun because you can do it any time you feel you need a good body stretch. Repeat twice daily.

Back Flexibility

Lie on your back on the floor with knees bent and feet flat on the floor. Raise hands toward the ceiling. Now move arms and turn the head to the right, while the knees move to the left. Reverse the above, then repeat. Gradually increase up to 5 and then 10 repetitions daily.

Bicycling

Lying on your back, move your feet and legs in the air as if you were riding a bicycle. Count to 6, and relax. Repeat, then gradually increase to 5, and then 10 repetitions once or twice daily if tolerated.

Elbow Stretch to Treat Tennis Elbow

With your arm extended straight out, parallel to the floor, lock your elbow and position your palm face up. Using your opposite hand, grab hold of the fingers and pull the palm of the extended hand toward the floor. Hold for 10 seconds.

Now do the same but have the palm facing down. Using the opposite hand, push the top of your extended fingers and hand down toward the floor. Hold for 10 seconds.

Hip Exercises

Flexion

These exercises are actually good not only for the hips but for the back and the knees. You can do these exercises on the floor or in bed.

Bend the left knee to the chest, and then bend the right knee to the chest. If needed, you can help by using your hands to help bend the knee. Repeat, alternating left and right knees. Try to increase to 5, then 10, and up to 20 repetitions, twice daily.

Pull both knees to the chest at the same time as in figure A.12. Hold this position for six seconds and then slowly rock from side to side while

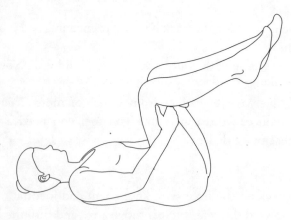

Figure A.12.

A hip flexion exercise.

holding the knees. Gently let your legs down. Repeat, gradually increasing to 5, then 10, and then 20 repetitions, twice daily.

Abduction

This can be done lying on the floor or in bed. While lying on your back (with knee straight or slightly bent), slide one leg out to the side, then return it to the starting position. Now do the same movement with the other leg. Gradually increase to 5, then 10, and then 20 repetitions for each leg, twice daily.

Extension

This can be done lying on your stomach on the floor or in bed. Keeping your knee straight, lift your left thigh straight up off the floor about eight inches (see figure A.13). Hold this position while you count to six. Repeat with the right leg, alternating the legs, and gradually increase to 5, then 10, and then 20 repetitions, twice daily. If there is severe pain, stop until you talk to your doctor.

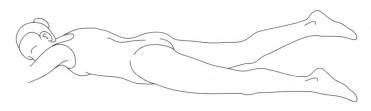

Figure A.13.

A hip extension exercise.

Rotation

Lie on your back on the floor or in bed. With your knees straight, turn your knees in and touch the toes of your feet together. Now turn the knees out. Repeat this, gradually increasing to 5, then 10, and then 20 repetitions, twice daily.

Knee and Leg Exercises

Extension

This exercise can strengthen the muscles of the thighs (quadriceps muscles), which offer major support for the knees. You can do this while reading, watching television, or riding in an airplane. The more you do it, the stronger the support for the knees.

While sitting in a chair, support your leg on a chair or table and straighten your knee as much as possible (see figure A.14). Then tighten your knee cap (push the knee down) until you feel the muscles of the thigh tighten. Keep that muscle tight and count to six. Relax, and then repeat, gradually increasing to 5, then 10, and then 15 repetitions, twice daily.

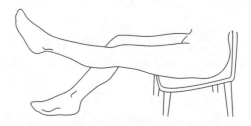

Figure A.14.

A knee and leg extension exercise.

Straight Leg Raise

While lying on the floor or in bed, bend one knee slightly with foot flat as shown, or bend the knee to the chest if you have chronic back pain. Raise the other leg slowly while keeping the back firmly on the floor or bed (see figure A.15). Raise your leg as high as you can, but stop if the

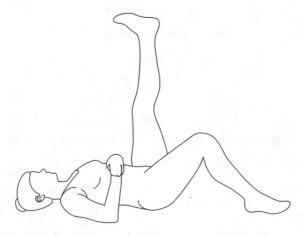

Figure A.15.

A straight leg raise.

back begins to arch. Hold and count to six. Lower your leg, and then repeat for the opposite leg. Repeat for both legs, gradually increasing to 5, then 10, and then 20 repetitions, twice daily. If you have severe pain with this or any exercise, stop immediately and talk to your doctor.

Flexion

You can do this on the floor or in bed. Lie on your stomach and bend your knees as far as you can toward your back. Straighten your knees, then repeat, gradually increasing to 5, then 10, and then 20 repetitions, twice daily.

Wrist, Hand, and Finger Exercises

Flexion and Extension for Wrists

With your arm on a table, counter, or chair, extend one hand over the edge of the table or chair. Use the other hand to bend the hand at the wrist up, then down as far as possible without pain (see figure A.16). Repeat, increasing up to 20 repetitions, twice daily.

Now placing your hand flat on a table, move the hand at the wrist so that your entire hand moves to the right, then to the left, as far as possible (see figure A.17). You can use the other hand for assistance if needed. Repeat, increasing up to 20 repetitions daily.

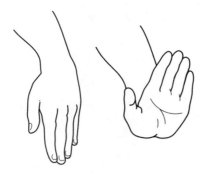

Figures A.16 and A.17.

Flexion and extension for the wrist.

Finger Flexion and Extension

Make a fist, then open and extend the fingers as straight as possible. Repeat this, gradually increasing up to 20 repetitions of each hand, twice daily. You can use a foam or a sponge ball (available at any toy store) about the size of a tennis ball to squeeze the fingers together. Release and extend the fingers.

Finger Curls
If your fingers are stiff, try to curl each finger down and bend each joint in the fingers as much as possible. Don't force the movement, but you can use the other hand to help curl the fingers of the first. Repeat and gradually increase up to 20 times for each finger, twice daily.

Finger Extension
Straighten each finger as you press the palm flat on the table. Don't force this movement if there is severe pain. This can be done twice daily.

Thumb and Finger
For grasp and pinch, try to form the letter O with your thumb and finger (see figure A.18). Make a good round O and then straighten the finger and move to the next finger. Repeat for each finger, gradually increasing up to 20 repetitions, twice daily.

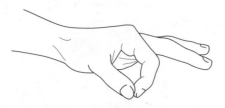

Figure A.18.

A thumb and finger exercise.

Finger Spreading
Spread the fingers wide apart, and then close them together as tightly as you can. Do this twice daily, increasing up to 20 repetitions each session.

Ankle and Foot Exercises
These exercises are easy to do and can be performed while seated almost anywhere. Raise your toes as high as you can with your heels on the floor (see figure A.19). Then press your toes to the floor and raise the heels as

high as you can see. Finally, rotate the ankles in a circle. Repeat each exercise, gradually increasing to 5, then 10, and then 20 of each one, twice daily.

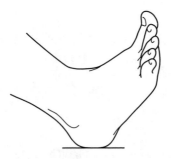

Figure A.19.

An ankle and foot exercise.

Resources

Research References

American Federation for Aging Research. "The Latest Research on Resistance Training and Aging." http://www.infoaging.org/l-exer-9-r-train.html. 2001..

Arnold, M., et al. "A randomized, placebo-controlled, double-blind, flexible-dose study of fluoxetine in the treatment of women with fibromyalgia." *American Journal of Medicine* 112 (15 February 2002): 191–97.

Arthritis Foundation. "Walking and Arthritis." http://www.arthritis.org. Accessed 18 October 2001.

Arts, S. E., H. H. Abu-Saad, G. D. Champion, et al. "Age-related response to lidocaine-prilocaine (EMLA) emulsion and effect of music distraction on the pain of intravenous cannulation." *Pediatrics* 93 (1994): 797–801.

Barbour, C. "Use of complementary and alternative treatments by individuals with fibromyalgia syndrome." *Journal of the American Academy of Nurse Practitioners* 12 (August 2000): 311–16.

Belch, J. J., et al. "Evening primrose oil and borage oil in rheumatologic conditions." *American Journal of Clinical Nutrition* 71 (January 2000): 352S–56S.

Benson, H., et al. "Relaxation Response: Bridge Between Psychiatry and Medicine." Medical Clinics of North America 61 (1997): 929–38.

Brewer, E. J., J. C. Bass, J. T. Cassidy, et al. "Criteria for the classification of juvenile rheumatoid arthritis." *Bulletin of Rheumatic Disease* 23 (1972): 712.

Bucsi, L., and G. Poor. "Efficacy and tolerability of oral chondroitin sulfate as a symptomatic slow-acting drug for osteoarthritis (SYSADOA) in the treatment of knee osteoarthritis." *Osteoarthritis Cartilage* 6 (1998): 31–36, Supplement A.

Cabral, D. A., P. N. Malleson, and R. E. Petty. "Spondyloarthropathies of childhood." *Pediatric Clinics of North America* 42 (1995): 1051.

Cassidy, J. T., and R. E. Petty. *Textbook of Pediatric Rheumatology*, 3rd ed. (Philadelphia: Saunders, 1995).

Castleman, M. *The Healing Herbs: The Ultimate Guide to the Curative Power of Nature's Medicines* (New York: Bantam Books, 1995), 27.

Cron, R. Q., S. Sharma, and D. D. Sherry. "Current treatment by United States and Canadian pediatric rheumatologists." *Journal of Rheumatology* 26 (1999): 2036–38.

Crosby, E. T. "The adult cervical spine: Implications for airway management." *Canadian Journal of Anesthesiology* 37 (1990): 77.

Cygan, R., and H. Waitzkin. "Stopping and restarting medications in the perioperative period." *Journal of General Internal Medicine* 2 (1987): 270.

Elkayam, O., S. Ben Itzhak, E. Avrahami, et al. "Multidisciplinary approach to chronic back pain: Prognostic elements of the outcome." *Clinical and Experimental Rheumatology* 14 (May–June 1996): 281–88.

Ferry, S., et al. "Carpal tunnel syndrome: A nested case-control study of risk factors in women." *American Journal of Epidemiology* 15 (2000): 566.

Fink, C. W. "Proposal for the development of classification criteria for idiopathic arthritides of childhood." *Journal of Rheumatology* 22 (1995): 1566.

Food and Drug Administration. "Overview of Dietary Supplements." http://www.cfsan.fda.gov. Accessed 31 October 2001.

Garfinkel, M. S., H. R. Schumacher Jr., A. Husain, et al. "Evaluation of a yoga-based regimen for treatment of osteoarthritis of the hands." *Journal of Rheumatology* 21 (1994): 2341–43.

Gavin, L. "Peri-operative management of the diabetic patient." *Endocrinology and Metabolism Clinics of North America* 21 (1992): 457.

Haber, D., and S. B. Goodman. "Total hip arthroplasty in juvenile chronic arthritis: A consecutive series." *Journal of Arthroplasty* 13 (1998): 259–65.

Hagglund, K. J., L. M. Schopp, K. R. Alberts, et al. "Predicting pain among children with juvenile rheumatoid arthritis." *Arthritis Care and Research* 8 (1995): 36–42.

Ilowite, N. T., G. A. Walco, and R. Pochaczevsky. "Assessment of pain in patients with juvenile rheumatoid arthritis: Relation between pain intensity and degree of joint inflammation." *Annals of the Rheumatic Diseases* 51 (1992): 343–46.

Jaworski, T. M., L. A. Bradley, L. W. Heck, et al. "Development of an observation method for assessing pain behaviors in children with juvenile rheumatoid arthritis." *Arthritis and Rheumatism* 38 (1995): 1142–51.

Jonas, W. B. "The effect of niacinamide on osteoarthritis: A pilot study." *Inflammatory Research* 45 (July 1996): 330–34.

Jones, T., and J. Isaacson. "Preoperative screening: What tests are necessary?" *Cleveland Clinic Journal of Medicine* 62 (1995): 374.

Komusi, T., T. Munroe, and M. Harth. "Radiologic review: The rheumatoid cervical spine." *Seminar of Arthritis and Rheumatism* 14 (1995): 187.

Kremer, J. M. "N-3 fatty acid supplements in rheumatoid arthritis." *American Journal of Clinical Nutrition* 71 (January 2000): 349S–51S.

Lan, C., J. S. Lai, S. Y. Chen, and M. K. Wong. "Tai chi chuan to improve muscular strength and endurance in elderly individuals: A pilot study." *Archives of Physical Medicine and Rehabilitation* 81 (2000): 604–7.

Love, P., and S. Santoro. "Anti-phospholipid antibodies: Anti-cardiolipin and a lupus anticoagulant in systemic lupus erythematosus (SLE) and non-SLE disorders: Prevalence and clinical significance." *Annals of Internal Medicine* 112 (1990): 682.

McAlindon, T. E., M. P. LaValley, J. P. Gulin, and D. T. Felson. "Glucosamine and chondroitin for treatment of osteoarthritis: A systematic quality assessment and meta-analysis." *Journal of the American Medical Association* 283 (2000): 1469–75.

McKechnie, A., F. Wilson, N. Watson, et al. "Anxiety states: A preliminary report on the value of connective tissue massage." *Journal of Psychosomatic Research* 27 (1983): 125–29.

Matti, M., and N. Sharrock. "Anesthesia on the rheumatoid patient." *Rheumatic Disease Clinics of North America* 24 (1998): 10.

Nierman, E., and K. Zakrzewski. "General medical care of the patient with rheumatic disease." *Rheumatic Disease Clinics of North America* 25 (3 August 1999): 585–622.

Pepmueller, P. H., and T. L. Moore. "Juvenile spondyoarthropathies." *Current Opinion in Rheumatology* 12 (2000): 269.

Reginster, J. Y., R. Deroisy, I. Paul, et al. "Glucosamine sulfate significantly reduces progression of knee osteoarthritis over three years: A large, randomized, placebo-controlled, double-blind, prospective trial." *Arthritis and Rheumatology* 42 (1999): 400S.

Reginster, J. Y., R. Deroisy, L. C. Rovati, et al. "Long-term effects of glucosamine sulphate on osteoarthritis progression: A randomized, placebo-controlled clinical trial." *Lancet* 357 (2001): 251–56.

Rooks, D. S., et al. "The effects of progressive strength training and aerobic exercise on muscle strength and cardiovascular fitness in women with fibromyalgia: A pilot study." *Arthritis and Rheumatism* 47 (February 2002): 22–28.

Smith, J. D., et al. "Relief of fibromyalgia symptoms following discontinuation of dietary excitotoxins." *Annals of Pharmacotherapy* 35 (June 2001): 702–6.

Svantesson, H., A. Akesson, K. Eberhardt, et al. "Prognosis in juvenile rheumatoid arthritis with systemic onset: A follow-up study." *Scandinavian Journal of Rheumatology* 12 (1983): 139.

Volker, D., P. Fitzgerald, G. Major, and M. Garg. "Efficacy of fish oil concentrate in the treatment of rheumatoid arthritis." *Journal of Rheumatology* 27 (2000): 2343–46.

Weintraub, M. 1992. "Shiatsu, Swedish muscle massage, and trigger point suppression in spinal pain syndrome." *American Massage Therapy Journal* 31 (1992): 99–109.

Wong, D. L., and C. M. Baker. "Pain in children: Comparison of assessment scales." *Pediatric Nursing* 14 (1998): 9–17.

Self-Help Products Websites

Accessibility Products Online
http://www.accesstoday.com

ADI Assistive Devices
http://www.geocel.com/adi/home.htm

Aids for Arthritis
http://www.aidsforarthritis.com

Comfort-Discovered
http://e-bility.com/comfort-discovered/arthritis.php

Comfort House
http://www.comforthouse.com

Dynamic Living
http://www.dynamic-living.com/alternatives.htm

Independent Living Products
http://www.ilp-online.com

Keyless Keyboards
http://www.keybowl.com

Life with Ease
http://www.lifewithease.com

Maddak, Inc.
http://www.maddak.com

Maxi Aids
http://www.maxiaids.com

North Coast Medical
http://www.ncmedical.com

Products for Senior
http://www.productsforseniors.com/arthritis_aids.htm

Sammons Preston
http://www.sammonspreston.com

Senior Shops
http://www.seniorshops.com/arthritis.html

The Boulevard
http://www.blvd.com

This company provides links to even more suppliers of self-help devices:
http://www.arthritis.org/resources/easy_to_use_products.asp

UK Websites

Arthritis Research Campaign
http://www.arc.org.uk

Arthritis UK
http://www.arthritis-uk.com

Arthritis Care
http://www.arthritiscare.org.uk

Arthritis.org
http://www.arthritis.org.uk

The Arthritic Association
http://www.arthriticassociation.org.uk

Children's Chronic Arthritis Society
http://www.ccaa.org.uk

National Rheumatoid Arthritis Society
http://www.rheumatoid.org

Worldwide Websites

Arthritis New Zealand
http://www.arthritis.org.nz

http://www.arthritis.co.nz

Arthritis Queensland
http://www.arthritis.org.au

Arthritis Foundation Western Australia
http://www.arthritiswa.org.au

Arthritis New South Wales
http://www.arthritisnsw.org.au

Arthritis Foundation South Africa
http://www.arthritis.org.sa

Index